ONE BODY

A Healing Ministry in Your Church

ONE BODY
A Healing Ministry in Your Church

DAVID ALDRIDGE

SPCK

First published in Great Britain 1987
SPCK
Holy Trinity Church
Marylebone Road
London NW1 4DU

British Library Cataloguing in Publication Data
Aldridge, David
One body: a healing ministry in your church
1. Spiritual healing
I. Title
615.8'52 BT732.5
ISBN 0-281-04324-8

Printed in Great Britain by
Latimer Trend & Company Ltd., Plymouth

To Felicity

Contents

Acknowledgements

The writing of this book was made possible by the love of my family, my friends and the parishioners of St George's Church, Wilton, Taunton. John Pritchard as our vicar, and friend, was instrumental in this work's beginning, and in its continuing. My good friends Laurie and Jenny Jeffery have sustained me and my family in times of doubt, and celebrated with us in times of joy. David and Elizabeth Spencer have supported us throughout the years when these ideas alternated between faith and folly. Patricia Smethurst ministered to me when I was in pain, and without her this work would have floundered. Bishop Morris and Anne Maddocks took me under their wing and gave me the necessary support and prayerful guidance which enabled me to go forward. Finally, this book would not have been written or this work fulfilled without the love, support and encouragement of my wife, Felicity.

Preface

This book is for leaders in the church community who want to motivate other members of their community to join in the process of healing. In many cases such leaders will be clergy who want to involve the laity in their ministry. However, lay leaders in the church community, nurses, hospital workers, social workers or doctors may also employ some of the approaches presented here. The book then is directed to 'carers' who wish to draw in other 'carers'.

Not everyone will want to do all that is written about here, nor will they have the resources. All that is asked of the reader is to consider some of the approaches and, when the time is ready, to try them out. The person who buys this book will probably have some ideas about beginning a healing ministry already, and the following chapters will give some practical help in realizing those ideas. The techniques described are intended for people who do not have a wealth of experience in community work, psychotherapy or healing.

When I talk of healing in this book I am using the word in the context of its etymological root of 'whole', 'healthy', 'holy'. Healing is a process, and a journey of discovery. It is not for me to offer a precise definition, for I do not have one. All I can do is suggest that to ask the question 'What is healing?' both promotes answers and raises yet more questions, while at the same time leading us to experiences of healing itself.

The journey

The model I have taken is the life of Christ. His injunction is to love one another, and the task is to 'Go out, teach and heal'. It is an activity demanded of all of us with the promise of guidance and of support.

While intended as a practical guide to healing this book is also about a personal journey with Christ. In my own journey into healing I have at times found that each daily happening has contributed to an experience of profound spiritual unrest. By living with this unrest I have also discovered times of great spiritual peace. Neither experience I believe is a whole by itself. It is the understanding of both together which is the Christian experience. The dynamic tension between the polarities of life – comfort and distress, loss and gain, living and dying – when embraced in the context of Christian experience, which has at its heart both the crucifixion and the resurrection, transforms our daily life. For me being a Christian is not an abstract entity or an intellectual pursuit; it is a living experience, an activity as vital as breathing.

Some people ask me about my faith, searching for qualities that I may have in terms of gifts, learning or intellect. I have no more such qualities than any other person. We are all alive, we have all been given the same promises by Christ. It is all too easy to look for the gifts of others and use them as an excuse not to act ourselves. Similarly we can all learn about the meaning of healing by acting in the world. Our understandings are negotiated and learned as a process. They are not delivered up to us on tablets of stone to live throughout perpetuity. The challenge for us today as Christians is to live, i.e. act, as Christians. Christianity is not the maintenance of a doctrine but an activity which takes place each and every minute of the day. For me the pursuit of healing is keeping Christ alive within me each day without submitting him to the suffering of Golgotha. And I fail. That is where healing takes place: in the struggling, the failing and the forgiveness.

This Christian life is above all an act of love. I have been most fortunate in my life, particularly in the past few years. I have been loved by many people. In that way I have received the love that many others feel to be lacking. This love had little to do with what I did; it was not a quality which I had, but one which was shown to me in many guises. This love for me has been a direct expression of God in the world. Love always sounds such a static word, as if it is some 'thing' which happens, and once having happened then remains the same or moves on to someone or something else. My experience has been something quite different. Love is an activity, perhaps better expressed as 'loving'. It is a process, it continues, and in its continuing I have discovered that God too is a process. God is the process at the very centre of my existence.

In this book you will find two contradictory messages. On the one hand I will appear to be saying 'This is how to go about healing'. On the other hand I am saying 'Ignore any doctrine; it is how you live your life, how you discover healing which is important'. Neither is true on its own. We all need guidelines and some structure initially, and the book is a response to requests for such structure. Yet I know that if the guidelines are seen as definitive then I have failed in my task. It is your understanding developing from what you do which is most important. Christ is to be found living in our hearts. It is in our daily lives when he lives again. We are his body. As we unite, as we reach out to touch each other, as we engage in the process of loving then he lives again.

Occasionally people who hear me speak say that it must be comforting to have a faith. My discoveries have been quite the opposite. In being human and a Christian the crucifixion is at the centre of my life. My life is therefore tragic and I am not spared tragedy. Any of you who begin a healing ministry must be prepared for this tragedy; otherwise healing simply becomes the ministration of a spiritual sedative. Once we accept the cross then we are allowed entry to the realm of redemption, the resurrection. We are offered a new life and we can have it now. Heaven is here, we can live in it if we act now. It is not a place to be found only beyond death but a corporate activity of which we can all partake. That is healing.

The structure of the book

The first chapter places healing as an activity which is being undertaken in a variety of contexts both within the Church and within secular organizations. There is also a brief account of how I came to be involved in healing as a Christian and as a research scientist.

The following chapters are concerned with the practical aspects of healing. My intention is that any reader should be able to dip into these chapters and have a clear idea of how to proceed after reading them. Not all of us have the opportunity to read all of a book at one go. This book, then, is rather like one of those gardening books which separates season from season and flowers from vegetables for the convenience of description. However, we know from experience that season follows season as part of a cycle, and that the separation of flowers from vegetables is an arbitrary distinction.

To extend this gardening metaphor further, Chapter 2 prepares the ground for a healing ministry. It deals with talking to the members of the congregation who may not share your initial vision. Unity is vital to the practice of healing. It would be to our shame if those practices we wished to introduce split our churches, and the pursuit of healing itself caused distress. This is not to say that there will not be struggle to introduce new ideas; rather that struggle can be creative and needs to be handled carefully. I shall also consider the relationship with complementary practitioners in this chapter.

Some church leaders ask me about healing and have a clear idea of the style of ministry they would like. They think of a particular style far removed from their own way of working and their own parish needs. Many people tell me of the marvellous ministries of John Wimber, David Watson, or Colin Urquhart. It is natural to want to repeat another's success. This desire for success is often based on a wish to serve. However, it is a trap. We cannot limit healing to a particular model. I hope at the end of this book that you will feel able to go out and begin a healing ministry. Certainly base your ministry on the same spiritual strength that inspires and inspired these individuals. Exercise that same trust in Christ, but allow Christ to work through you. The ministry of those who do this will differ according to the persons involved and the type of parish. There will of course be some common elements but the practice will be particular to the needs of those whom you serve.

Chapter 3 is concerned with the use of meditation. Meditation is used in this sense as a particular structured activity for healing. There are practical examples for composing your own 'meditations' using biblical themes: for individuals, for families, in home groups and in worship. My own practice uses meditation for the relief of pain, for relaxation, for releasing our own inner resources, and for listening to God.

Chapter 4 describes the formal sacraments of healing, the laying on of hands and anointing with oil in the context of healing services. The practical issues of organizing the service are covered here. We cannot divorce healing from the other activities of the Church. Healing is located within the context of praise and worship. As the reader will notice throughout the chapters, healing is placed within differing contexts and adapted to those particular needs. My fear is that healing will be treated as a separate activity. I believe that it should be practised in a natural manner and be part of our natural Christian activity. In our worship we give glory to the Lord. It is in this giving glory that we become united. In this unity we become whole: although we are many we become one body. And that is healing.

Chapter 5 extends this work to the use of the formal sacraments of healing within the home. A significant part of my work is concerned with home visiting and the use of healing with individuals and frequently their families and friends. Part of this chapter will describe the way that some structure is introduced into these home visits.

Chapter 6 links the previous activities together and focuses on a community approach to working with families. This chapter deals with neighbourliness, befrienders, and the development of home-visiting teams. Most people will see this as no different from the practice of pastoral care. I would not argue with that. What I urge you to do is to engage in as many practices of care as possible so that healing is seen in as many areas of church and community life as is possible.

A major foundation of any healing ministry is an active prayer life. Not only is this fundamental to our faith but allows for many people to be involved and to play a part. In my work non-Christians are turning to the healing ministry for help. The offer to pray for and with those persons is an example of our love. I find that their willingness to accept prayer is a sign both of their awareness of spiritual needs and of God's grace for all people. The more I work in this way the more I see that to divide the world into Christian and non-Christian is a most un-Christlike activity.

To unite these activities I will present some examples of working with people who have encountered cancer. Real-life stories always personalize what are inevitably abstract descriptions. Many issues will be raised by these accounts about the nature of healing and about suffering. My understandings are still partial. It is not with any sense of modesty that I say 'the more I know the less I know'.

Those of you who do embark upon a healing ministry will find continually that deep and profound theological and existential questions will be raised. These questions will be provoked by the very activity itself. They will come from others with whom you work but often from deep within yourself. These questions are very important. Healing is a process. It is not a separate activity which we do to others. It is an act of living faith of which we partake in the company of others. The metaphor for this process, which runs like a thread through this book, is that of a journey. Some parts of this journey undertaken with others are described in Chapter 7.

The final chapter discusses the need for spiritual direction for those involved in the healing ministry. I also introduce the concept of the wounded healer and the need to examine our own prejudices and assumptions once we begin upon this journey. It is all too easy to be apparently willing to serve others and yet be unaware of our own needs which are being met in that service. Finally, I discuss our relationship as members of a healing endeavour with other complementary practitioners and alternative medicine.

1 *A Journey into Healing*

Healing is a current issue. Each year there appear to be more and more books about healing and whenever I speak to individuals and groups they tell me of the books they have read and urge me to read them too. The majority of books about healing fall into two broad categories. One group is the abstract theological discussion of 'healing' within the modern Church. Abstract discussions leave us asking the question 'Well, what do we do?' The other group is that of individual witness and personal ministry. Both have their place, yet both leave a gap. Personal witness all too often leaves us feeling either helplessly inadequate or spiritually inspired and wondering what on earth we can do. My concern is that spiritual inspiration from personal witness is fine *if* it is turned into healing activity. All too often the closing of the book signals the closing of the endeavour. While we discuss theological niceties, and in some ways indulge ourselves with inspiring stories, people suffer, members of our own communities live in isolation and much of the world starves.

Healing as activity

In this book I will propose ways of beginning and developing a healing ministry within your local church. Many of the theological arguments will be taken for granted. They are not dismissed. The assumption is that by the time you have reached the point of using this book you will have already become acquainted with the theological background to Christian healing or have decided to introduce a ministry of healing.

In a local survey of churches from differing traditions I discovered an active interest in healing on the part of the clergy. Their main need was in the area of pastoral counselling, particularly from a biblical or Christian perspective. Although chronic physical illness was seen as the main focus for sacramental healing, mental illness was regarded as the target for counselling. The problems of chronic depression, alcoholism and also severely debilitating mental illness were concerning priests who felt unable to meet the needs of their parishioners who had such problems. This was emphasized by a corresponding concern about the burden of care being shifted from the hospitals to the community without consultation, and principally, adequate resources.

My personal belief is that some theological insights are best based on practice. What appears to be theoretically adequate within the context of a group discussion or even in a book is quite different in practice. In my own work I have found that ministering to the dying within the context of a healing ministry has meant a deeper understanding of healing and of living. This is perhaps a reversal of the usual practice whereby religious practice develops out of theology. I am advocating the exercise of compassion in practical acts as a Christian activity first, and suggest that theological understanding will develop from those acts.

You are not being asked in this book to surrender your doubts, if you have any. What I am suggesting is that in the very act of 'doing' questions are answered and some doubts are dispelled. In my clinical practice I often ask people to maintain their doubts while at the same time venturing out to try something new. In this way the old is not discarded but becomes transformed in the light of the new. Truth is something which we determine and discover. It is in the activity of ministering to others where the real debate about healing takes place. In reading this book you will find areas where we both agree and disagree. I make no claim to any authority of truth. All I ask is that the ministry begins where compassion holds sway over rhetoric and love reigns over dogma.

Some of what you read in this book you will be doing already as part of your work in the community, as part of your sacramental ministry, or in the day-to-day activity of parish life. Hopefully the suggestions in the following pages will be seen as building on what you have already, rather than tearing down and starting afresh. My position is that we start with what we have and move on from there. It is important that we, as experts, do not indirectly 'de-skill' those with whom we work. Our parishes are full of latent talent. I hope that in the following pages you will feel that those talents can be developed and used to the full.

A concern of some priests is that we can become too organized and that an umbrella organization of a healing ministry can prove restrictive. My hope is that this book will allow church communities to pursue their own initiatives to meet their own needs. My belief is that in the long run church communities with different traditions will feel free enough to unite in their healing endeavours. In this way individual differences are celebrated but in a context of united practice to meet the needs of the wider community.

By insisting on maintaining our traditional beliefs and practices in their purity we do not allow ourselves to be open to the changes demanded of us. Unity at a deep level means that we must die to self (even the 'self' of an institution) and become new. In this way the old order dies to become renewed in Christ. Too often our efforts at unity are superficial. We conspire to co-operate with just enough effort to avoid the challenge of deep commitment and change. Although we may make gestures to satisfy our desire for unity, those gestures without deep commitment can conspire to keep us apart and 'unchanging'.

Healing as a journey

In the eighteenth century the explorers who set out paid heed to the 'rutters' or *routiers* of their navigators. These were the maps and charts of little known areas of the seas. Their purpose was to point out difficult waters and likely areas of danger. In some ways this book is a *routier*. In it you will find practical descriptions – charts if you like – of how a healing ministry was set up in an active church community. There is no intention that this book should be a definitive description of how such a ministry is carried out. That, I believe, would be wrong.

Not only will this be a voyage of discovery for your church community, it will also be a personal voyage for you. There will be times of joy. Many of you will already have had the experience of seeing people recover from illness or tragedy and healed. At the same time ours is a faith which encompasses both joy and sorrow. There will be times when we cannot hide from our own spiritual poverty, when we cannot hide from the death of Christ. This too is part of the same voyage. Only by accepting both sorrow and joy can we make our voyages those of discovery. This requires a firmness of will. To venture into healing requires a spiritual sturdiness which itself is gained during the journey.

I learned early in my voyage that a desire to serve does not itself mean that this desire will be met. At times we are becalmed. After reading about healing, practising healing, writing and publishing papers both here and throughout America and Europe I expected to be invited out to august gatherings where healers gathered together. It was a long time before anything did happen. During that time all sorts of questions and self-doubts arose. This is an important process which I now call consolidation. At the time I was both angry and impatient to begin.

Wanting to be used is the first step. There is no guarantee that you will be used or used in the way that you think best. Any endeavour which involves our personal vision is inevitably limited. By insisting upon our vision we can blind ourselves to the wider possibilities of healing. I have had the pleasure recently of working with two men who are eminent in their respective fields of practice. Both decided to unite on a project which would bring about what they most desired. However, in the planning stages there were real difficulties. The negotiation of a co-operative endeavour meant both of them had to face the loss of part of what they cherished most as individuals to gain what they most desired as a team. Our cherished desires are partial; as soon as we begin to work with others then we cannot do exactly as we wish. Furthermore we have to learn that in the working through of conflict and the negotiation of co-operation then healing begins to take place. In this way as Christians we offer the world practical examples of alternative resolutions of conflict.

Know your community

There is as yet no template for healing ministries. How your healing ministry turns out is up to you and your collective endeavours to suit your church community. I know this will not suit some people who want clear solutions to all their problems. What I shall be proposing is a means of resolving issues and a way of proceeding. Of course there will be concrete steps to take. However, do not believe that these steps are the only ones. My hope is that you will see what I propose and then take this proposition and act in your own way.

The working out of solutions which 'fit' your community is part of the process of healing. Externally applied solutions are never as ecologically sound as internally developed solutions. Although these internal solutions demand patience and co-operation, precious gifts in such hurried times, they are always pertinent to the needs of those being served. External solutions are often partial and bring their own problems. We know from the aid given to third-world countries that external aid is only effective as an emergency measure. The real aid comes in developing internal solutions.

In some ways this way of working reflects a modern concern in medicine. People are being urged to take charge of their own health. There is a move away from the separation of the body from the mind and the spirit. With the prevalence of persistent chronic illness, the continuing presence of cancer and heart disease, modern technological medicine is being found wanting. Mechanistic notions are being abandoned in favour of holistic models. The physician is seen as setting the scene for healing to take place rather than being the agent of that healing. At the same time we are beginning to question the authority of doctors in deciding our health concerns.

Similarly within the Church there is a movement to involve church communities in the recognition of a common priesthood. The Church is beginning to see that the life of the community is the responsibility of the whole community acting together. In our modern communities we are at a crossroads. Authority is being questioned. This is not to deny the professional expertise of doctors and priests, but to use them in a different way: as facilitators and guides. It is to respect their advice and use their expertise within a framework of communal responsibility where we all begin to take responsibility for ourselves and others.

To act in this way means moving from a position of curing and being 'cured', from the signs and wonders of modern medicine or powerful individual ministries, to a collective act of healing where we take responsibility for the health of the community. I am not suggesting that modern medicine or individual healing ministries be displaced: rather that we shift our emphasis from the short-term and temporary measures to long-term understandings and changes in practice. While it is important to carry out emergency procedures on a person who has had a heart attack it is also important to consider the lifestyle of that person. If that person continues to smoke heavily, drink half a bottle of whisky a day, is about to become redundant from a job and lives in a situation of extreme marital and familial stress, then short-term solutions will never achieve a long-term resolution.

By the same token, while it is important to maintain and promote individual endeavours, and the sacramental administration of healing, it is also vital that we locate these acts within a corporate ministry of healing endeavour. People often ask me to see their family or friends and lay on hands. My response is to ask them what is preventing them from laying on hands, or anointing with oil or praying? I possess no gifts which they do not have access to. Similarly it is the same God who hears and answers their prayers, the same Spirit who guides them. Throughout this book my position will always be that 'You can do these things. You can reach out and touch. You can pray. You can exercise compassion'. What I urge you to do is to begin the process of healing. Do not set your hearts upon a grand ministry but be confident that your ministry will develop its own shape. The process of healing is not passive. As you go forward then be continually open to influence. Listen and learn from others with whom you are in contact. Not only will you find that your ministry flourishes but that you change too. You will be taught what works.

Healing as a social process

Scientific medicine has come under considerable attack recently. One area of criticism has been the neglect of the person and the continuing focus on technology. Another criticism is that technological medicine has been unable to address certain aspects of chronic degenerative disease, e.g. arthritis. Scientific medicine has continually played down the relationship between social factors and ill-health, but more significantly has neglected the whole area of health-care delivery. The delivery of health care is a process involving many people who interact one with another. The whole process of becoming ill, of choosing self-care remedies or deciding when to consult a practitioner is a social process. When we become ill few of us do so in isolation. What symptoms signify 'illness' are negotiated within the context of those with whom we live our daily lives. What to do about those symptoms depends upon many different factors. This is the context of popular or lay health care.

For instance we may develop the symptoms of 'flu. Our spouse will presumably apply the appropriate home medications and allow us to be free of domestic responsibilities temporarily. However, should we extend the symptoms overlong, or make a miraculous recovery when a friend calls on us to go out socially, then our 'illness' may become seriously questioned. Popular health-care practice is important and we have only a limited knowledge of what happens. Most episodes of illness are treated or managed at home without seeking any outside help. Of equal importance is the process whereby we decide that home-care remedies are inefficient and that we need to contact external help. This process involves decisions about whom to consult: i.e. do we see our family doctor, do we see a 'healer', do we contact a 'counsellor', or do we look for an alternative or complementary practitioner? It may appear straightforward to some of us that as soon as we decide that a problem is acute then we contact our family doctor. This is not a universal practice. Many people who have chronic problems with pain or arthritis are likely to use a range of differing practitioners.

The development of 'holistic' medicine and 'alternative' therapies has attempted to redress this balance. Alternative, or complementary medicine, advocates the integration of body, mind and spirit. Health is not merely the presence of physical signs and symptoms but a *relationship* between the state of a person's mind and the body's functioning, and that person's sense of connection to a spiritual realm. At last there is a growing awareness that people in despair become sick.

A difficulty of this approach is that these different realms of understanding – the physical, the psychological, the spiritual, the cultural and the philosophical – all depend upon differing means of validation and explanation. Their common feature is that they all reject the crude materialism of scientific medicine which relies upon measuring things which are countable and discrete. Scientific medicine is interested in *disease* which is somatic and belongs to a rational theoretical structure.

Complementary practitioners are more concerned with *illness* which belongs to the realm of personal experience and meaning. However, once we leave this realm of what is concrete and countable then we have to rely upon less satisfactory evidence. Similarly these therapies emphasize the connection between the practitioner and the patient in the healing encounter. Patients are not merely objects which are 'done to' but are equal persons involved in a process of healing. Professionalization has often meant the distancing of patients from practitioners. By giving priority to the disease then the person becomes lost.

My concern is that we should not be too ready to dismiss scientific medicine. What we have to do is to integrate scientific medicine into the practice of health-care delivery. This means changing our whole societal perspective from a passive acceptance of health care, or to be more accurate illness care, to that of active health initiatives. As communities we must engage in those activities which promote health. Similarly we must engage ourselves in the debate about what counts as health. Once we begin to do this then we move away from narrow concerns solely about our own health and consider those connections within our family, within our community, within society and within the world.

Family medicine has begun to make some headway. Some symptoms are seen in the broader context of the family and social network. There is a rising concern for the health of the poor and the unemployed and their children. This concern is also mirrored in consideration of the presence of marital and relational conflicts and the incidence of poor health. What we need to do is to offer practical initiatives which reach out to meet those concerns. General practitioners may have the understanding that social, spiritual and relational factors are involved, but they do not have the resources to deal with those factors.

Our task is to meet those needs in a working relationship with the general practice of family medicine. I do not promise that it will be easy. To embark upon such a process is a political move. The shift of emphasis is on the communal exercise of primary health care. It is a move which will emphasize our personal rights and our social obligations for the health of those with whom we live.

The care practised in the health centre is only one facet of our health lives. In the same way church services are only one aspect of our spiritual lives. These practices are important, but they are only part of the greater context in which we live our lives. Although we rely upon our priests for guidance it is we who must be responsible for our spirituality. In the same way we must become responsible for our own health. Further to this I believe that we must become responsible for our own health together. When we do this, healing becomes the centre of our health activities. Healing becomes a ministering to one another. Our relationships become therapeutic.

Who is to heal?

Healing in the Church has been an issue which has challenged authority since its very beginning. Each time healing has come to the fore it has raised fundamental issues of both belief and practice. However, although the issues have been raised there has been no cumulative response to healing which has been developed into a universally accepted practice.

It seems that healing becomes an issue during times of change and unrest within society when people begin to demand a respite from their suffering, when social disorganization threatens personal integrity of body, mind or spirit and injustice is evident. We have such a situation today. Our society is divided. There is poverty throughout the country of both spiritual will and material need. Terrorism and threat are a common currency with violent act matching violent act. It is we as Christians who must begin to heal divisions and minister to these needs. This ministry is not restricted solely to those of us who have university degrees or specialist training. The emphasis we place upon literary skills and educational attainment acts as a form of licensing which restricts the activity of our parishioners. The call to the disciples was to follow Christ. No demands were made of them to establish their intellectual or social credibility. Patience, faithfulness and love are qualities which we can all exhibit and it is perhaps these credentials we should seek.

I will continually refer to the need for the Church and medicine to unite in meeting the health needs of our communities. Yet the unity of these two institutions is only part of the picture. If healing remains the concern solely of those two institutions and neglects to involve the lay community then nothing will change. The twin hierarchies will simply combine to maintain the practice of expert elites ministering to what they believe is the need of others. Similarly we must beware of becoming 'healers' who are recognized as experts and inhibit the healing activities of others in the community either by practice or reputation. In my visits to see various healing traditions I have been dismayed to see large congregations who have venerated individual healers at the expense of developing their own healing initiatives. We must not allow the gifts of individuals to inhibit the development of gifts within the body of the Church.

What we must do is to listen to the needs of all the community. Then we must use the skills resident in the community. Our position as experts remains the same, yet we advise and consult, co-operate and facilitate. In doing this we help our communities to recognize their own health needs and develop their own healing gifts and initiatives. The outcome of such endeavours is that crises are avoided and self-help is promoted.

A personal journey

Occasionally I ask myself: 'How did I manage to get caught up in all this anyway?' This usually happens before I have to give a talk at a conference, or am about to address an audience that is hostile to the idea of healing.

Most of my early career was spent working with young people. As a teacher and youth worker I came to be interested in those young people for whom a youth service was offered, but who somehow never used this service or saw it as relevant to their needs.

In the early 1970s there were the first inklings of youth unemployment. Even at that time the poorly educated found difficulty in finding employment. Those young people who had been in prison or borstal faced even greater problems. It was to these young people that I directed my work. Similarly there was a group of young people who had family backgrounds which were unsupportive. They had little opportunity to develop or express themselves. They were often in trouble with the police and had no parental support. With these too I chose to work.

Once I began to work with these young people I found that acceptance was the key to meeting them as persons despite our personal and social differences. I am not ignoring the fact that patience would have been a useful gift too, but if patience is a fruit of the Spirit I had a succession of poor personal harvests during those years. Many of the young people I worked with had been systematically demoralized. Their voices were unheard. They were inarticulate verbally yet articulate in their despair.

Given the chance to communicate, to ask without being disparaged, to be valued, then they began to value themselves. It was during this time that I began to understand the necessity of working with families.

Although I saw individuals and groups of young people, whenever someone turned to me in distress it was not that person only who was distressed but also the people with whom they lived. The more I worked with juvenile offenders and young men who were in and out of prison the more often I found that they had families who too had needs which were unmet. They did have the support of the social services and the probation service but the administration of social welfare singularly failed to meet their needs as 'whole' persons. The satisfaction of material need was present but there was little provision for emotional and spiritual support. A major difficulty was that these people were outcasts and deviants even within the realms of social service. They were seen as difficult people to deal with, as 'unfortunates', as not worth bothering with.

The more I dealt with individual suffering the more I found that their loved ones suffered too. When a young man was imprisoned he often left behind a young wife and child. This woman and child were often abandoned by their own family for marrying too young. Where then was the caring in a Christian society?

After this time I moved with my wife and family to Cornwall. While studying for a social work qualification I wrote my first thesis on the occurrence of suicidal behaviour in families and how to work with people who had attempted suicide. This was based upon my work with Samaritans, but principally from a research project which followed up one hundred people who were discharged from a general hospital. The more I worked with the suicidal the more I became appalled that nothing was being done to help the despairing.

Since the early 1960s there has been a massive increase in the number of people, particularly young people, who intentionally overdose or injure themselves. Some commentators suggest that this is unlikely to diminish in the near future. Deliberate self-poisoning has become the most common reason for the acute medical admission of women to hospital and poses a major challenge to health-care services. For men, deliberate self-poisoning is second only to heart attacks as the most common reason for admission to hospital. Much of the published work which dealt with the suicidal described the suicidal person as deviant and suggested that there was little which could be done therapeutically to help. The notion of prevention had all but been abandoned in the medical and psychiatric literature. Suicidal behaviour was seen as a uniquely individual and impulsive act.

This was unacceptable to me. People become suicidal. If we look at their circumstances we see that the situation in which they live begins to deteriorate. I set out to understand these processes of becoming suicidal particularly in the context of family relationships. Fortunately after a lot of writing around to universities a grant was made available for me to study for a doctorate in the department of psychology at the Open University.

While researching into the occurrence of suicidal behaviour in families I came across a group of people who had become suicidal after a history of chronic pain. No matter what they had attempted the pain had failed to go. A suicide attempt usually took place after their general practitioner and a series of consultants could find nothing physically wrong with them. They were seen as difficult patients. Their problems were thought of as psychological. The attempt at suicide was considered as yet another piece of evidence that they were manipulative and difficult rather than sick and despairing.

A colleague and I decided to work with these so-called difficult patients. We used all our collective counselling and psychological skills and set about learning more. Before each patient and their family came into the interview room I would spend time being quiet, becoming still, praying for that patient and preparing to listen. I shall cover this area in a later chapter. One of my concerns about counsellor training is that a lot of emphasis is placed upon active skills with insufficient emphasis on preparation.

Somehow, people began to get better. There were spontaneous recoveries. In the broader work with suicidal families fewer people repeated episodes of suicidal behaviour and those who came to us feeling suicidal were helped. By seeing people in the context of their family relationships then the ground where they had become suicidal was covered. A feature which distinguished families where suicidal behaviour was present from those where suicidal behaviour was absent was the presence of three variables. First, the family or marital relationship was about to split up. Second, everything anyone tried to do in these families was seen as being wrong. Thirdly, the person who became suicidal had a history of becoming sick at a time of conflict in the family. Becoming sick was a way of averting a family conflict which, it was feared, would tear the relationship apart. This fear, which was often quite false, was the very factor which prevented some families from changing.

When this research came to an end some members of our church community, our priest, my wife and myself decided to concentrate on using our energies to pursue a full-time ministry of healing within our local church. A year before we had spent a residential weekend away with the parish talking about 'wholeness'. I discovered that the meditation, relaxation and touch that I used with patients were similar to the activities that other Christians were talking about as acts of healing. Rather than merely continue talking about a ministry of healing we decided to do something. One of the first things I did was to go and see

Bishop Morris Maddocks who invited my wife and myself to join the apostolate of the Acorn Trust. Later he came to our church and held the first in a series of healing services.

That local ministry has developed. It is that development which is described in the following chapters.

2 *Introducing Healing to the Church Community*

After hearing about healing, and understanding how important it is, it is rather tempting to demand a ministry within your church community. Unfortunately this approach may generate as much hostility as it does enthusiasm. It is very easy to be enthusiastic oneself and then blame others for their lack of your zeal!

If healing is to take off and to endure then it is vitally important to involve as many of the church community as possible. There will be some people with whom you will actively struggle. Cherish them and listen to them; they will teach you many things. I am not advocating that you become less enthusiastic or change your beliefs in any way, but rather that you use all the resources of the church to bring healing.

It is best to use the particular style which your own church practises to get across important information. Whatever you do make sure that your bishop, or if you are a lay leader, your vicar, and the church elders are aware of your intentions and that they support you. There is no point in trying to carry out a ministry of healing if the result is to split the church community. If the parish is such that lay initiatives are not listened to, or implemented, then the first step is not a formal healing ministry. The first step is to develop a forum whereby lay ideas are listened to. Therein lies the healing, the wholeness between clergy and laity.

There are various ways of directing attention to healing. Talk to each other, and more importantly listen to each other. Once you embark upon the step of launching an idea as a project it ceases to be yours. It is important to present some examples of what the ministry would entail in terms of services, in the use of buildings, in the allocation of funds and also who would be involved. It is often a good idea to bring in an outsider at this stage to give a 'one off' talk. That person will take some of the heat off you and you can be critical of them and propose ways in which you could do it differently. Sometimes hearing ideas spoken by a third party gives you sufficient distance to understand others' objections to those ideas, or even to hear the ideas anew and be revitalized.

Attend as many courses and meetings as you can about healing and immerse yourself in the literature. No doubt you will have read about healing and possibly have been to a meeting already. Actively seek out practitioners from other traditions and see what they have to offer. Now is the time to expand your own knowledge. Similarly it is essential to grasp the biblical teachings about Christ's healing work. Nobody expects you to become an expert. In some ways it is important to allow others to have expertise to complement your knowledge. What you must have is a grasp of the breadth of possibilities and a confidence in your own knowledge when you answer questions. There is nothing wrong in 'not knowing'. It is, however, important to be aware.

Then you should go out and talk to established groups within your church. Introduce them to healing. The main thrust of the work is to place the idea of healing firmly within the culture of the community. Once the idea is being talked about then the practice can follow. Somewhere the spark of enthusiasm will start a fire of support. These talks will certainly test your ingenuity.

The principal consideration is to talk in the style of the particular group. If they regularly have activities then introduce healing prayers as an activity. If the group like to sit back and be lectured to then give your best lecture using carefully prepared notes.

Talking to groups

My way of working with groups is to engage them in talking to each other fairly early on. The format I use is outlined below.

(1) Start with a time of worship and prayer. Involve those to whom you are introducing the idea of healing. It is important right from the start to get across the notion that healing is an activity within the compass of all those present and that you expect others to join in. Most of all it should be fun and enjoyable. It is a shame if we make healing an activity separate from the rest of the activities of the church. Healing must be embraced within the framework of worship and praise. Worship opens our hearts to celebration and is an important preparation for healing.

I would go even further and say that the healing lies not solely in the formal or specific healing activities themselves but in the whole context of worship and healing. It would be a pity if in our search for wholeness we became partial in our practice.

(2) Say who you are and what you do. If you are a parish priest then perhaps this will be obvious, but it is an opportunity to present a brief picture of the breadth of your work. If you are in a leadership role within the church or your local community tell the group briefly how you came to be interested in healing.

We like to hear about the person who is talking to us. It is not simply curiosity but an activity which allows human beings to identify the understandings which they share. Similarly, by telling about ourselves people realize that we have no special qualities to which they cannot have access.

Certainly we have all had varying experiences and have developed different skills. However, none of us has any monopoly of spiritual gifts or of grace. I challenge people to dismiss any thoughts that they cannot do any of the things which I talk about. We are all given the same promise by Christ that we can go out in his name and do what he demands. Furthermore, he promised us that the Holy Spirit would be with us to guide us. Note that there was no restriction of this guidance to people with degrees, to men only, or to those with the ability to speak. A challenge we all face as Christians is 'how can we all be involved in healing?', for we all must surely pursue unity.

Healing is an activity concerned with our very vulnerability and the essence of our humanity.

Allow approximately ten minutes to tell the group about yourself.

(3) Divide the large group up into smaller groups and appoint a spokesperson for each group. If the main group is only small then allow people to find a partner. Make sure that you have some sheets of paper, a blackboard, or an overhead projector on which to write down any answers to your questions. The reason for doing this is that people are far more likely to take on board information and ideas, if they have been involved in the process of talking about the ideas and understand the ramifications of those ideas in practice. Then ask some or all of the following series of questions. Pause between each question. Allow time for discussion and debate. Sit in on groups and encourage people to have their say. After the allotted time – again about ten minutes – get the groups to report back what they have said. Restrict them to two sentences to each group but allow all to have their say. This restriction promotes the notion that all can participate while discouraging the person who always wants to get up and make a protracted speech.

Ensure that all persons say to each other that they will respect each other's confidences and that it is important *not* to say anything if they are at all hesitant about doing so. It is important to allow people to feel safe. Many issues are difficult to express. Take time to establish a relationship of trust first. Then people will not feel that they have blurted out something personal, or that they appeared foolish.

Before each question is asked allow a few minutes of silent contemplation for the groups to quieten themselves and focus on the activity.

(a) What are your expectations of the day? It is important to make sure that you meet the needs of the group you are speaking to. Recently I ran a day workshop with a friend who belongs to our church community and has been active in the healing ministry. She came with me to pray, to offer support and to talk informally to conference delegates and answer some of their questions. During the first session, after the worship, when expectations were elicited she noticed that a man in her discussion group repeatedly mentioned the need for personal physical healing. Later in the day she was able to pray with this man and his wife which brought them both comfort.

This personal need was in contrast to the other needs of the group. The important consideration was that all the needs of the group could be stated and some attempt be made to meet them. These needs were wide ranging.

For example, some people came along to sit, relax and listen openly to what was being said, simply allowing themselves to be receptive. Others came along wanting to know about self-help activities in which they could engage. Others wanted guidelines about beginning a healing ministry within their church. Yet others wanted to know how to cope with the feeling of being drained after listening to others in difficulty or distress. Some wanted to know about the notion of holistic medicine and links with 'alternative' or 'complementary' practitioners. Some wanted to know if people were 'born' healers and others were simply seeking inner peace.

As the reader can see there are enough expectations there to last more than one day! What I did was to introduce the guidelines you will find in this book, to address all of the expectations and discuss some of them briefly, and introduce some relaxation exercises and meditations.

The most important activity is to give people the chance to express their needs vocally, and to discuss them with each other. It is a model for how the healing ministry can begin in a church. Get people together to state their needs. Allow an open expression of those needs and begin to address them. Some can be addressed immediately using your own knowledge. Other needs can be met by community expertise, i.e. what others know. Some needs will not be met immediately, but once expressed there can be a plan to set about meeting them.

It is important to use the expertise of others and thereby involve them. To involve others removes one person from taking on sole responsibility and becoming identified as the 'healer' or the one person responsible for the healing ministry. This is not to abdicate responsibility. One person can be co-ordinator, but it is important that the message goes out that 'healing' is a communal activity in which all members of the church can play their part.

After this session take a break to sing and pray. It is useful after any period of concentrated activity to have a break. In this way people have some time to take in what they have understood and heard consciously and subconsciously. By refraining from thinking directly about what has gone on before, we allow ourselves time to assimilate what we have learned. Much of what we learn goes on out of the range of our conscious understanding. Having said all that, any one who knows me personally will tell you that a chance to sing on any pretext will be taken up! Once again celebration is fun, we open our hearts and give access to those parts of us which are emotional as well as intellectual. It is all too easy to talk about love and forget that it is essentially an activity.

Now is a good time too to have a break for tea or coffee. This will give others a chance to continue informal discussion and for you to make sure that you can meet most of the expectations of the people who are there. If you cannot meet some, then say so. It may be a matter of too little time and you can arrange to talk again at a later date or propose a series of meetings. Some expectations I cannot meet and have to say so. I find it difficult to come face to face with some theological questions in a way which is intellectually satisfying for the questioner. There is no harm in not knowing. The challenge is for the questioner. By taking everything on ourselves we actively inhibit the ministry of others. A healing ministry is about the sharing of gifts, developing those gifts and promoting those gifts in others. Similarly, for some people direct answers are the wrong solution. We underestimate the value of finding out. I don't know a lot about healing, but what I have set out to do throughout my life is to discover all I can about it, in the company of others, guided by Christ. It is important that by giving seemingly definitive answers we do not inhibit the same process in others. Discovery is not about 'answers' but the continuing process of questioning.

(b) Why heal? This question immediately addresses the theological issues involved. With each church group with whom I have done this so far, there has been a broad spectrum of reasons both within the groups and within churches. The very activity of discussion is important. People within a church begin to raise arguments which are fundamental to their systems of belief.

The liveliness of debate imbues the healing ministry with a vitality. Somehow the core issue of Christ being active in the world is raised. Our faith is related directly to important and concrete issues and individuals are given the opportunity to do something. Rather than be demoralized by events which seem out of the control of the individual, people are encouraged to apply their Christian faith to real issues in their daily lives.

(c) Share your experiences of healing with those in your group. Take it in turns to speak to each other. It is important to witness to healing in all forms. I encourage people to talk about hospital treatments which have worked too. It is important that we do not set aside the work of hospital doctors and general practitioners as being separate. My intention is to encourage others to see the hand of God in all healing, not to restrict healing to those activities which are pursued solely by healing ministries.

After this witness, there follows a time of quiet. Each person is asked to bring into their mind's eye someone they know who has been healed, or who is in the process of being healed (all of us). A prayer of thanksgiving is then said.

(d) What healing activities do you participate in already? It is important to emphasize that healing is not a strange and separate activity. Many people already pray for the sick, visit the needy and counsel the distressed. If we emphasize competence and existing ability then we build upon an existing foundation. We also give out the message that we are recognizing the competence of others and are not the sole possessors of some idiosyncratic and special gift.

(e) What inhibits the healing ministry within the Church? All too often people say they cannot do this or that activity within a church because it is not allowed. In this session it is important to be positive and to suggest ways of working which encourage hope and co-operation. For those who are isolated in their ministry it is important to link them with another person either from within their own community or with someone from another church, so that they may pray together. The important part of this approach is to insist that there is no one template for the healing ministry. It will vary and it is important that we do vary what we do.

Our ministries must meet the needs of our communities; they cannot be imposed upon them. For those who have tried already to start a healing ministry it is important to emphasize persistence, to keep on asking to receive, or to keep on knocking until the door is opened. It is important to spend some time after this session praying for obstacles to be removed both from within ourselves and from within our communities. There can be a time when people are allowed to pray spontaneously and voice their own obstacles, and a time of silent contemplation. I usually introduce a meditation at this point where we imagine the light of Christ permeating all situations and dissolving all obstacles as the tide smooths out the sand on the seashore.

(f) What do you see as the main contribution that your church community could make towards healing in the area where you live? This session gives the opportunity to formulate concrete goals. It is a move from abstraction and obstruction towards positive planning identified in particular activities in specific situations. Before any talking begins have ten minutes of silence and allow thoughts to emerge. Emphasize that this is a time of 'no thinking' but of 'listening' and 'receiving'.

Get people to be specific about what could be done, encourage them to formulate specific goals. It is important that these goals are attainable. Rather than embark upon some massive visionary programme it may be more appropriate to begin with something quite small. I am not being unduly pessimistic here. All too often we only hear of marvellous schemes which are impressive and have great prestige. Perhaps it is time we began to marvel at the myriad small miracles which take place all the time. Perhaps the foundation of modest initiatives will allow us all to unite in a common shared endeavour.

Now take a time to celebrate and pray. A time of thankfulness for our own abilities is appropriate here, then prayers for guidance in achieving the goals that are described.

(g) How can the Church and medicine be encouraged to work together in your local community? Whom could you encourage? What activities would they engage in? Once more allow some time to be silent and for answers to emerge. This process means that we do not have to leap into answering questions straight away. By making a link between the Church and medicine we are linking two institutions which have similar aims. Many of us have doctors among our parishioners – perhaps it is time to make plans to talk to them about how we can share in our communal health endeavours. Where there are hospitals then there are chaplains and there are possibilities for supporting them. When people are discharged from hospital there is necessity for support. While people are in hospital there are families who need help. However, above all there is a real need to meet the spiritual requirements of those who are in distress. Our spiritual needs are part of our total 'health'. It is to no avail if we try to medicate for depression if the person concerned is lonely and feels abandoned by God, is in the process of divorcing a spouse, or is about to be made redundant from work and drinking half a bottle of whisky a day.

Before the next section take a break for a song if possible. If this is not appropriate then talk about a particular aspect of healing which interests you. This enables you to break up the pattern of the activity for a while. Another way would be to stop for a tea break! Remember to fit into the style of the group of people to whom you are talking.

In this following section it is important to reassure those present that you are not going to ask them to do anything strange or untoward. Ask the group to sit quietly with their eyes closed for a period of ten seconds, breathing deeply. Then to open their eyes. That is step one. Step two is to ask them to reach out for the people to the left and right of them if they are sitting close together and to hold them lightly on the lower arm. You are going to ask no more of them than that. Say that it may be initially embarrassing but you believe that they will overcome this. Ask them to release their touch and ask the following related questions.

(h) What do you believe needs to be healed:
- (i) in the world;
- (ii) in the community;
- (iii) in the church;
- (iv) in your family or close relationship;
- (v) in you?

After each subsection ask the group to close their eyes, reach out to touch each other and for one person or all of the group to pray for those issues which they recognize need to be healed. As you will see the questions become more specific. It is up to you which questions you choose to ask or not to ask on the grounds of appropriateness or time. Ideally you will formulate your own questions.

A weekend away

In our church the healing ministry was focused at its very beginning by a parish weekend away together. A group of us went away to Abbey House in Glastonbury. There we spent a weekend talking about, praying for and meditating upon 'wholeness'. This format of extended discussion, worship and prayer is an ideal foundation from which to build a corporate ministry. It is thus possible to discover a wide range of talents and involve others in making plans, with a time to consider the ramifications of current and future commitments.

Home groups

In our church it was the home groups which provided the nurturing ground for the healing ministry. These groups are held fortnightly in the home of a parishioner. They are lay led either by individuals or by pairs. While being ideal places for teaching and debate they are immensely valuable for nurturing relationships and introducing new people into the church community. I will discuss these groups later in the book.

Their primary function in the context of this chapter is as a forum for the introduction of healing. Before my involvement some of the groups had used audiotapes obtained from the Lee Abbey community at Lynton in North Devon as a guide to talking about healing. After our parish weekend away where healing was discussed I began a four-part series of sessions using meditation as an introduction to healing. After these experimental sessions we would discuss healing as an activity within the Church. The discussions were broad and wide-ranging, covering the biblical aspects of Christ's healing, and extending to the place of healing within the context of modern medicine. This series of sessions was repeated at other home groups. Some people came along specifically to learn about meditation, others came to discuss healing. The principal effect was to introduce into the church community an active debate about healing, with active considerations of what could be done.

From these home groups people have asked for healing or have felt that they could attend a healing service. One of the difficulties that we have found is that people see healing as some form of magic, and wonder how on earth such a ministry could apply to them. It is by speaking in the security of the home group, with the opportunity to ask questions without fear of embarrassment or condemnation, that people begin to hear the truth about healing. Significantly the meaning of healing is negotiated between people who are intimately connected with each other. What is said is only part of the activity. Communication involves more than the words we speak. We give out messages in the tone of our voice and by the posture of our body.

When people are given the chance to voice their doubts then we are given the chance to learn. By listening to the concern of others about healing, particularly the confusion of healing with curing, then I have learned to present material in a clearer manner. However, beyond all this, when we attend to each other with careful listening then we are giving out a powerful message. We recognize the worth of the other person. We engage the other person to seek the truth with us.

Magazines

If you have a church magazine, either write a regular article about healing and the issues it raises yourself, or invite a parishioner who has experienced healing to contribute. Similarly you, or a member of the church community, can write a regular review of books concerned with healing. A doctor in the parish may want to raise an issue involved with his or her work as a Christian and a short article in the magazine is a useful vehicle for such comments. New material spreads the word further and continually keeps the idea of healing in the forefront of the church culture.

It is also useful to collect personal testimonies of healing and present these in a magazine or journal. For example: a parishioner wrote about her visit to a morning service and how she had experienced the healing love of Christ in the singing of the music group. Another person wrote in the magazine of her gratitude for the support and friendship she had received at a time of difficulty. Do not restrict yourself to physical healing, look for examples of reconciliation and comfort at a time of loss. All too often we restrict our understanding of healing by being far too narrow. Once we adopt a notion of 'wholeness' then we begin to see many examples in our daily lives of rifts being healed, growth where there was once sterility, and peace in place of strife.

Summary

Teaching is an active part of the healing ministry. Healing is introduced within the culture of the church. This teaching is best done at a number of differing levels: through written material, through the spoken word to large groups, through direct experience, by individual spiritual direction and within the context of intimate home groups. The overriding concern is to find the most appropriate conditions under which people will learn. If we take care to nurture the soil and provide the appropriate climate then the seed which is already sown will spring into life.

3 *Meditation and Healing*

A significant part of my work uses meditation. I need a time of peace and quiet to listen to God. When working with others I introduce a means of listening which allows them to become still. When we reach times of crisis in our lives we can all too easily fuss or panic and so compound our difficulties. At other times we can be paralysed by anxiety, not knowing what to do next. The stillness of meditation, where we can allow ourselves to be filled with God and experience the thrill of being enlivened by the Creator, is a wonderful song in our spiritual repertoire.

All too often we use our prayer life to throw demands at God after busily rushing into activity. We are eager to serve yet unable to listen to his voice. In this way prayer becomes a means of telling God what he should be doing if he were half as wise as we, rather than meeting the true challenge of the co-operative partnership he offers us in the whole of creation.

In meditation we take the route of the contemplative which is to discern what it is that we need to pray for and to hear Christ praying within us. In the latter part of this chapter I will introduce you to such meditation. This need not restrict the reader to the style used here – it is possible to use other meditations from within the Christian tradition. The techniques discussed can be learned and implemented by anyone who is interested in the church community. In practice this has been either clergy or home group leaders who are already in a role of leadership in the Church.

The first stage of meditation involves relaxation. Many people come to the groups I run to learn this technique of relaxing as a relief from stress. Although relaxation is an important factor in the process of meditating the process I describe will not be simply and solely a mechanical technique. Occasionally meditation is criticized because it appears to be secular in terms of techniques and also for the part relaxation plays in those techniques. In my clinical practice I am involved with teaching and researching stress-management techniques and the practice of self-care. I know that the spiritual, the psychological, the physical and the social cannot be separated. People ask what to do and how to do it. We can use techniques and remain aware that there are other dimensions of awareness involved. This is not meditating by numbers, although I will use a technique of counting to provide a structure in a later example.

My intention is to give people the means to enhance their listening to God. At the same time they can gain some relief from the stress of daily life, discover the source of healing within themselves and find a haven of quietness deep within them. That involves learning a technique. To be a brilliant musician requires many abilities, one of which is a highly developed technique. The same applies to our spiritual discipline: we need to develop our repertoire of skills. As long as we remember that skills and techniques are only part of the necessary requirements then we will keep them in balance.

This way of working is primarily about becoming still. It can lead people to discern the appropriate action to take concerning a particular problem. Rather than running around in circles jumping to the old conclusions and getting into a greater muddle, meditation allows people to sit quietly and allows solutions to emerge. Invariably these solutions are the most appropriate solution for the person. First, they are not those applied by an outsider. Second, they use the full problem-solving capacity of the person. This emphasizes that the person is capable of solving problems. Third, understandings and solutions are reached calmly, quietly and in the context of Christian listening. In terms of healing we contact the source of healing which is the fount of all wisdom, God within us.

In my work I prefer people to discover their own solutions. Such solutions are always far more suitable than those I might suggest to them. Rather than listen to me they listen to God. The metaphor I try to use is that of a personal ecology: what a person does has to fit into the ecology of their personal relationships, with their personality and into a particular culture. In this way people do not become dependent upon me as a therapist or as a guide. They learn to develop the skills by which they can discern the guidance of God.

Meditation is an activity that must be practised regularly. Somehow people come to expect immediate grace or some instant magical transformation to a state of deep peace. Although this way of working can bring immediate benefit it is important to explain that it has to be worked at. We would not expect to pick up a musical instrument and play untutored. Similarly with meditation it is important to gain some tuition and, above all, to practise.

I hope this does not put any one off meditation. The whole process is as easy as breathing and needs only a little applied imagination. What it amounts to is a waiting on God, listening for the word to be spoken, for the image to be revealed or for the knowledge to be discerned. I use the three modes of sight, sound and knowing because people experience their spiritual understandings in different ways. If we listen to people talk, some people will say 'Do you see what I mean?', or 'Does this sound right to you?', or 'I knew this would happen'. This is not purely a figure of speech. The way we talk about the world reflects the way we experience the world. Similarly we reflect our experience of God.

In the following meditation you will see (even hear or know) how I structure the meditation using and invoking a variety of senses. This is to develop as many possible channels of experiencing stillness and as many possible ways to 'hear' God. The full development of our internal sensory world leads us to wholeness.

My main aim throughout the meditations is to lead the person meditating to a direct encounter with God. This is not for me to mediate in. I am only a guide. The experience of being in the presence of the living God, of being made whole by Christ, of listening to his voice can only be known by the person meditating. I hope that you can learn how to be a guide yourself both from these words and by regular practice.

The notion behind this means of working is that Jesus Christ is risen and lives today and speaks to us. We can enter into a dialogue with the living God. All of us, not just professionals whether priests or psychologists, who struggle to listen with a desire to hear will hear. How we hear, as I have said earlier, differs. Some of us do hear words, others see pictures, yet others feel the touch, and others simply know.

Sometimes I am asked if meditation is rather a self-centred activity akin to the idea of contemplating one's own navel. I can see how this misconception occurs as many of our images of people meditating are generated from pictures of people sitting in the lotus position, or of composure in the middle of a crisis. My reply is that meditation is, in the end, activity-centred. It should lead to action in the world, but not activity for activity's sake. Some people become very active Christians: they are visibly, and often audibly, 'busy'. However this may be of little use and may be pursuing either wrong action, or right action in the wrong direction. If we are so busy that we become discouraged, or as the current jargon says 'burnt out', then we have acted wrongly. How often do we see church leaders dashing from one crisis to another, plugging the gaps without stopping to check if the plugs are appropriate?

Meditation in the way it is used here gives the opportunity for quiet contemplation, to allow what is deep to emerge from beneath the superficial. In my life meditation leads me to ways of reconciling conflict. First I begin to understand where the conflict lies in the relationship without blaming the other person. Then, second, I place this relationship before Christ and see what he has to say to me or to the other person, and what is the next appropriate step to take. This link between what is understood in meditation and action in outward life is what turns the process into meditation rather than vain imagining.

In the same way when I work clinically with families, couples or individuals I will ask them to take their conflict to Christ in a meditation and ask for forgiveness, or direction, or healing and see what Christ does. They can then translate such an understanding into action in their daily life. This is a very private way of working too. Those people who do not feel they can articulate their difficulty, or that it is too embarrassing, can be helped without divulging anything to another person. They can confess to Christ and see an appropriate resolution for their problem given the appropriate guidance.

Getting ready to meditate

I will describe the process I have used in the home groups mentioned in Chapter 2. First we talk about any important issues which need to be raised and make sure that anyone who has anything they are burning to say can say it. Second, prayers are said. These can be prayers of spontaneous welcome, particular prayers for the season or the collect for that week.

If a new group is involved I will spend some time explaining who I am and what I do. Then I will say what meditation is. I will also tell people that they will not have to sit or lie in any strange position and that they will not be open to any external suggestion. For groups where a person is wary of meditation and not sure of the approach but still wishes to try I will introduce a prayer of protection asking Jesus to surround us with his light.

Meditation can be practised anywhere once the person is well versed in the technique. However, for the home groups the place is usually a room in a house. People are asked to sit with their hands in their laps, with their legs uncrossed and their feet flat on the floor. It is not essential to have hard straightbacked chairs but they are the best. Not only does this stop people drifting off to sleep but stresses the importance of still attentiveness. Although in meditation we become relaxed and quiet we also become sensitively attentive.

Once everyone is sitting comfortably I ask them to leave the cares of the day behind and to be prepared to learn something for themselves which will be of use. It may be that they learn that they do not wish to pursue meditation. If that is the case then they can be sure that truly entering into the process will give them the basis for a decision. For those with a particular problem I ask them to release it temporarily with the promise that they will be able to recall it later in the meditation in a different way. This means of learning involves sitting quietly and not trying too hard. Perhaps the best way of learning!

The meditation: the light of Christ

The following pages contain the transcript of a meditation which took place in the house of a friend. The meditation was one of a series of four which were used in the context of a home group to introduce Christian healing to our church community. The transcript contains descriptions throughout of the technique I am using, and why. You can use this and adapt it as you wish. My main intention is that you have some idea of what a constructed meditation looks like.

The full text was not written down before I started simply because I had practised and used this meditation many times with other groups. However, I do change the timing and content according to the people present and the way in which they respond during the process. This is an interactive process which takes notice of the people present. All that you have to do is to take your time, watch for the clues that people are becoming quieter, and then continue.

As in all aspects of the healing ministry it is important to know the people you are working with and fit whatever you are doing to meet their style of worship and understanding.

This meditation would be preceded by a welcoming prayer.

If anyone is wearing contact lenses it is a good idea to remove them before starting.

> *Allow your eyes to close. If you wish to fidget or move, feel free to do so. If you want to cough, then cough.*
> *Be aware of your breathing, don't try and do anything about it at all, just be aware of your breathing.* (*20*)

As you can see I have introduced a number, 20. I will introduce a number at regular intervals throughout the meditation. There are several reasons for this. First, with the gradual reduction in the number from 20 to 1 then the person can discern, in the context of a new technique, that which is familiar. Second, the use of a number promotes the idea of stages. These stages can be those of moving down or of deepening. Third, the use of numbers is a part of a later technique whereby people can reach a state of meditative quietness using a ritual of counting down. This is not overly psychological. We all use the same process when we sit in our seat in church. We are going through a ritual which leads to a state of awareness. The countdown technique is particularly important for use in the relief of pain, for sleeplessness or in times of crisis. I will discuss this at the end of the chapter.

You will also see that I use the term 'allow' throughout the meditation. This is to emphasize the voluntary nature of the method. I cannot induce anyone to do this beyond their own volition.

The emphasis on breathing is deliberate. Many studies have been made of the effectiveness of deep-breathing techniques upon our bodily systems. It is vital not to ignore this. Breathing is a natural activity and encourages in the person the sense of security that they can begin with something that they are capable of. I would like to add here that, although breathing is a natural activity, we sometimes do adopt and sustain breathing techniques which are downright harmful. By being aware of our breathing we begin to breathe slowly and deeply.

The recurrent demand is to 'be aware'. I am not trying to lull anyone into a state of unawareness but to help them to focus their own awareness. Our bodies are continually feeding us information, most of which we ignore. Occasionally we need to attend to that which we are ignoring. In the process of becoming aware then we begin to know ourselves and beyond the knowledge of our bodies we begin to know God.

At the same time be aware of the natural sounds of the world around you, that wealth of natural sound, and the sounds beyond those sounds, the sound of the distant streets. (*19*)

Allow yourself to become comfortable, to fidget or to move,
allow those movements to discharge themselves through you
and be amused that as soon as you start to become quiet
you begin to move,
and be attentive of those sounds within yourself, (*18*)
the sensation of your heart beating,
the sensation of your tongue within your teeth,
the sensation of dryness within your throat. (*17*)

In this section the person is being encouraged to listen to the messages of their own body. All too often we ignore the natural signs our body sends us. The process of meditation is one of attentiveness focused on a particular area of our consciousness. In the first few lines I ask the person to focus on external sounds. As soon as we become quiet then we begin to hear the new tapestry of sound which the world makes. Paradoxically, silence is noisy.

Moving from external sounds to internal sounds serves two purposes. First, the person focuses inwardly. This also helps to avoid any distractions from other people in the room who move or cough. Second, when some people become quiet they experience their own bodily sensations. For some people these commonplace experiences seem quite unique. The expression of those sensations allows them to understand that nothing strange is going on and further stresses the natural process of becoming still.

It is important to let people move freely. Becoming still initially involves movement. Sometimes people try to hold themselves completely still. This is counterproductive as they fail to relax sufficiently.

As you breathe allow yourself to breathe in as if you were breathing in light, and allow that light to spread into your shoulders, into your chest,
allow that light to enter into you,
and as you breathe in allow that light to spread through you,
through your shoulders and down through your arms,
through your hands and through your fingers.
Allow that light to pass down through your body, through into your hips,
down through your legs, (*16*)
down through your ankles and through your feet, and allow that tide of

light to pass through you. (*15*)
As you sit or stand by the shore as the tide comes in,
the relentless tide which spreads further and further,
allow that tide of light to wash over you and through you,
allow that tide of light to flow over and through your hair,
and relax,
and through and over your eyes,
allow the tensions to drain away,
and down through your cheeks,
and through your mouth,
and relax.
and through your jaw,
and allow yourself to become heavier,
and relax,
Allow that tide of light that washes over you and through you to wash through your shoulders and through your chest, down through your body, through your legs, through your feet. (*14*)

This is a straightforward relaxation technique. It also introduces the person to the use of imagery in the process of meditation by talking about light. The use of light is deliberate for it is in the process of 'breathing in' Christ, the light of the world, that we become enlightened. I do not say directly during the meditation that we are breathing in Christ. I allow people to make whatever connections they wish during the process.

Note also that we can change meanings here from 'breathing in' Christ, an inspiration, to a breathing 'in Christ' where we breathe as a body held by Christ.

It is important to understand that, although this appears as a uniform procedure, many people will experience it differently. Some people say that I miss particular numbers out. Others do not even notice that I count! This further emphasizes that communication is a collaborative process involving both the sender of the message and the listener. We can propose all manner of things but they need to be heard correctly. I occasionally find that people take offence at what I say when no offence is given. The process then is located within the listener who 'takes' offence. In the process of meditation we not only develop passivity, but also, an active listening.

Imagine any problems you have, no matter how small,
imagine them as piles of sand,
as if we had them by the seashore.
Find them by yourself and make them into piles of sand,
and just as those relentless tides by the sea wash away those piles of sand and erode them,
allow those same piles of sand to be dissolved by that relentless tide of light

which passes through you.
Allow those problems to be eroded by that tide of light.
It may be a problem you have in a part of your body,
it may be a problem you have in the things which you think,
it may be some worry,
allow that tide of light to wash over and through it,
allow those problems to dissolve,
you will still remain as a person,
you can exist without your problem, (*13*)
and as that tide of light washes over and through you
allow yourself to become deeper and deeper,
and relax,
become quieter, allow that remorseless and relentless tide to pass over and through you.

The use of imagery is developed further here and directly applies to a particular problem. As the reader will see, repetition plays a vital part in the technique. What a written account cannot do is to demonstrate how I allow my voice to become slightly deeper and slower as relaxation becomes deeper and quieter. Do not hurry through this process. You can speak much slower than in conversation, with regular pauses. When talking about tides it is important to allow that sweep of the tide to be in your voice.

Pay great attention to the people you are working with. Notice how people look and sound as they become relaxed. Their whole body posture changes. Synchronize your speech with these changes. Similarly notice how their skin tone changes and how they begin to breathe diaphragmatically (literally deeper). We are not separate from the people we work with. I like to imagine that in these classes I am engaged in a beautiful and graceful dance with the people in the room, our minds and bodies linked together in co-operative movement. Or that we are singing a song of praise together, each solo voice distinct but fitting into a common song which is eternally singing within us, at times in unison and at times in harmony.

Be aware, on the one hand, of whatever sensations of comfort you wish to have, and allow that to happen.
Be aware, on the other hand, (*12*)
of whatever levels of relaxation you wish to have within you.
Be aware of a third experience, you say that you wish to experience some healing,
and be curious about what experience of healing you will have. (*11*)

By locating recognizable sensations in either hand then people are allowed to have both comfort and relaxation. They are also being directed to focus on whatever levels they wish to experience, which puts those experiences within the abilities of their own bodies. At the same time they are given a third proposition which is slightly confusing. They have 'no hands' logically to consider healing on, but they do have the body between to experience healing in. They are asked to be curious about what healing will occur. Note that I do not say 'if'. My understanding is that healing is a continuous process. All I am asking the person to do is to discover this process in whatever way they can. This may be at any level and it is important that I do not limit the person's understanding of healing.

As that tide of light passes over and through you,
down through your face,
in through your jaw,
through your chest, through your hips,
through your legs, and through your ankles
imagine the person on your left also sitting in that same tide of light
which passes over and through them,
and imagine them presenting those problems which they cannot always find for themselves,
allow them to discover those reluctant problems they have,
and allow them to dissolve those reluctant problems as relentless as the tide on the shore. (*10*)
Be aware that you both sit in that same tide of light which washes over and through you,
and be aware of that person on your right, (*9*)
of that tide of light which passes over and through them and experience them becoming deeper and quieter,
how you both share that same light which washes over and through you, (*8*)
and as we all sit together in that same tide of light which washes over and through us
allow that tide to dissolve those problems which we keep close within ourselves,
which we are reluctant to release. (*7*)
Although we are many we share that same light. (*6*)

As you can see, the major premise underlying this section is that of 'though we are many, we are one body'. Sometimes people feel that to spend time upon themselves, and to care for themselves, is wrong and selfish. By allowing themselves to see others enveloped in this same light, which they share, then they can see what change looks like. If we can observe healing in others then we can begin to contemplate our own healing. When we witness healing, no matter how small it seems to us, then we are witnessing the emergence of the Kingdom of God. There is a danger in any ministry, I believe, that we minister only to others and neglect ourselves and pretend that this is self-sacrifice. By doing this we hide our own imperfections, content to seek the failures of others and ignore our own weaknesses. All too often people try to become therapists to meet their own needs of completeness.

Imagine if you will that you see a stained glass window in all its colour,
and its form, its beauty and its meaning,
you are that window,
allow yourselves to be seen,
watch yourselves being that window,
be that window. (*5*)
Be aware of the light beyond,
the light which brings that window to life,
and through that window that light is seen, (*4*)
allow that tide of light to wash over and through you as you become deeper and deeper, (*3*)
and prepared for any experiences you may wish to have, (2)
you become quiet, and peaceful, within yourself. (*1*)

By asking a person to see themselves in the context of meditation then we are asking metaphorically for them to stand outside themselves. I use this part, but elaborated to a greater degree, in the management of pain. If we ask a person to step outside of themselves temporarily then we can give them the opportunity to consider themselves in a different way. When a person is in pain I will ask them to see themselves separate from their body where the pain is located and to make sure that that body is comfortable and free from pain. For others I may ask them to see themselves lit by the light which passes through the window and see what understandings emerge. If we pursue understandings which emerge from illness then we realize that all aspects of our lives have the possibility to enlighten and transform us.

The pursuit of only one form of active health is not only a rejection of the disabled but a crude form of materialism in itself. By pursuing norms of health rather than understandings of health and illness then we invalidate and disable others far beyond their physical incapacities.

Stay at whatever level of awareness you wish to have, whatever you need for yourself,
there are some things you may wish to know now and experience them,
and if you wish you can also conceal them from yourself,
and that is all right.
Some things you may wish to understand but not to know, and conceal those things from yourself.

This is an injunction used for one purpose only and that is for people to learn about achieving a level of relaxation or stillness. The reason I ask people to conceal understandings from themselves if they wish is so that they do not have to rush off and consider how to use this knowledge. Similarly the relationship between understanding at a deep level and knowing at a conscious level are separated. By doing this we can learn to trust our inner resources. Some psychoanalysts have emphasized the unconscious as a primitive force deep within us which often appears as chaotic, impulsive and archaic. I believe that this negative view of the unconscious is misguided. Within us we have a deep and broad knowledge which does not conform to the constrained knowledge of our conscious logic. This knowledge is timeless. It is located in the pattern which connects us within the universe to all that is. That knowledge is God emerging in us. The unconscious then can be an important creative and unifying force within us. In his book *Steps to an Ecology of Mind* (Paladin 1973) Gregory Bateson reminds us that 'the heart has reasons which the reason cannot know'.

I'm going to ask you to go to a quiet place within yourself,
a place to which you can go at any time,
a place you know deep within yourself,
and I'm going to ask you to count down to there.
While I am counting down you may find yourself that instead of going down you may wish to go up,
and there may be no steps, merely a path, and although I ask you to go through a door, for some of you it maybe a gate and for some of you you may just pass through, do not be concerned with my words, alter these experiences to however they will work for you. (*5*)
Be still and at peace within yourself, not having to do anything.
Being aware but not busy, (*4*)
and allow yourself to make any commitments you may wish to make, (*3*)
or any understandings you may wish to find. (*2*)
Be prepared to go to that quiet place within yourself. (*1*)
And enter into that quiet place.

Finding a quiet place within ourselves is essential for our spiritual peace. Rather than locate peace outside ourselves we can find an internal haven of our own. This understanding can be used at times in our lives when we need to use meditation in a different way, either at a time of crisis, or when we need to listen carefully to God. For those of us who travel on crowded public transport or work in a busy office then a haven of peace is our own chapel.

By asking people to adapt these words they are encouraged to use the words creatively. Sometimes people say that the words were not quite right, or an image did not fit. With practice and skill we learn to guide people with greater finesse. However, it is far more important that we encourage people to take responsibility for themselves. Creativity is within the grasp of all who listen. The use of the images, door and gate, is important. Jesus says 'I am the Way'. These images are another invitation to discover the way within us.

While you are there light a candle for yourself,
and another candle for someone you love, for those you love,
or those that are close to you,
and bring those candles together.
See how those candles are separate but how the light they give out merges together.
We are the candles, God is the light.
In this quiet place be prepared for whatever experience of God you wish to have here,
whether it is a sense of awe,
or a sense of deep peace,
or reverence.
Some people find the very presence of Jesus.
He puts his arm around you and holds you like a lamb.
Allow yourself to be comforted,
to be restored,
to be quietened.
For some of you who may wish to try this,
if there is someone who is close to you who perhaps you are arguing with,
imagine them in this quiet place, allow them to come closer,
and within the presence of Jesus,
allow yourselves to say the things you need to say,
allow yourself to say those words of forgiveness,
and you may ask for help.
By the same token,
allow yourself to hear those same things back from that person,
allow yourselves too, to be forgiven.
Imagine what it would be like,
there may be things you wish to say which have gone unsaid over the days or over the years, things which should have been said,
allow them to be said in the presence of Jesus.
This is the process that you can do at any time
and be comforted.

This passage speaks for itself. Forgiveness is fundamental to healing. In all aspects of my work I come across the need for forgiveness. Time after time the anger of bereavement and the despair of loss can be transformed after years by asking for forgiveness. I encourage people to enter into a dialogue with others, to practise a dialogue within their hearts, to rehearse forgiveness. In this way they can go out into their active lives in a different way. Either they say something to the other person and ask forgiveness, or more importantly they live their life in a different way. By using a time during meditation then we go beyond words and the limits of our habitual behaviour into the realms of active compassion.

I am going to ask you now
within that quiet place within yourself,
to discover a spring, a source,
a fount of healing within yourself.
Some people find a spring,
some find a rushing torrent, some merely a hint,
but in God's presence
allow that source of healing to spread within you.
Imagine that you could allow that healing to grow greater and spread to another part of your body.
I wonder if you could get it as far as your shoulders,
or even as far as your elbow,
or down even as far as the tips of your fingers.
Or even that source of healing down through your body,
down through your ankles, down through to the tips of your toes,
or even that source of healing within you that could stretch through your jaw, through your skin, right through to the inside of your scalp,
and just imagine how with God's help that source of healing within you can fill you full to every pore,
through every cell.
You can be bathed through every internal part.
Imagine that this internal source within you could spread beyond you, until it became bigger,
until it became an aura around you.
Breathe in the Spirit to assist you.
As you breathe in the Spirit allow this aura to grow stronger and stronger,
and extend this aura to the person on your left and allow them to be made whole.
And extend this aura to the person on your right,
and allow them to be made whole.
Allow them to be healed and comforted.
While you are breathing in the Spirit bring into this aura of healing those in the congregation at church,
those in your family, those who may be ever so far away,
or those who may be very very close.
Bring them within that aura,
see them as they would be healed,
or well,

how they would be active; laughing, being.
Allow that aura to envelop them, and realize that you can do the same things for yourself.

As the reader can see in the above section, healing is located within the person and extended to others in the group. When this is done in a group all involved are part of a communal experience of healing. From this position it is possible to go out into the world and heal filled with the knowledge of the Spirit within you. By experiencing this process of healing as a flow within you it is possible to work actively towards healing without words, simply by being. When we become filled to overflowing with love then we enter into healing relationships. Consider the implications for yourself and a group you meet with regularly if you sat and practised this method! As an experiment try filling yourself in this way before you meet someone you argue with, or before a difficult meeting. Maintain that experience of deep peace and fullness of the Spirit. Be aware then of any changes in that relationship. If you are struggling with someone try taking that relationship to that quiet place within yourself and use Christ within you as a consultant. Ask his advice. Hear his words.

I am going to ask you to leave this quiet place within yourself in a moment.
Be aware of this quiet place,
that you can have access at any time,
that the door itself will open,
that this place is always there within you,
that this source of healing always flows,
that it is within you and without you, there eternally.

First I am preparing the people present for a change when I tell them what is to happen in a moment. As a technique in the construction of a meditation the use of a statement to prepare the listener is a means of punctuating a change and giving them a chance to be ready. While they wait it is possible to reinforce the experience of the quiet place within and that it can be returned to and used at any time.

Allow yourself to leave this quiet place.
I am going to count now, (*1*)
and I am going to ask you to imagine, on one hand,
that you are a river bank, the one side firm, secure,
the rock, the soil, the vegetation, rich, fertile, (*2*)
and, on the other hand,
you are the other bank of the river,
whether new or old,
made of sturdy materials
whether concrete, clay or stone built,
constructed soundly, secure.

Between each side flows a river
a source, a continual flow.
You are not sure where it begins or where it ends, (3)
but on each side and on each bank you experience that flow,
and each bank contains the river, (4)
yet, at the same time, you know
the river forms the banks, (5)
determines the shapes of the banks, (6)
the banks shape the river, (7)
the river shapes the banks,
and just as you imagine each side of that river,
experience that constant flow,
on the surface, what appear to be two sides,
deeper, at the bed of the river,
both sides join together. (8)
What at the surface seems like two separate things
deeper are one, (9)
and allow yourself to understand
that we are all different banks,
and we all share that same river. (10)

All religions use healing metaphors. Jesus told parables as a form of instruction. By using stories and metaphors we provide people with enough information for them to make their own sense of things. Understanding is an activity. In this instance it is one of promoting unity out of difference. Disparate states, two different banks, are united at a deeper level, the river bed. Similarly we can be led to understand the interaction of both the bank and the river, each constraining or influencing the other.

In my clinical work with people who have had long-standing problems I regularly use metaphors and stories. Indirectly we can talk in a way which is beyond the limitations of our formal logical language. By invoking images of health, growth and relationship in a story we foster the context for people to enter into that alternate reality. In this way we change. As Jesus knew, a story draws the person in and actively involves their imagination.

Allow yourself a feeling of refreshment,
a feeling of joy
and of restoration. (11)
That you have had certain experiences you may wish to conceal from yourself, (12)
and certain experiences (13)
you may wish to discover at a later date.
Allow yourself to be refreshed, (14)

as if you are standing by a cold lake in the mountains
or you are drinking a cool glass of water. (*15*)
Or you are standing by the seashore
with the mist on your face. (*16*)
Allow yourself to be restored
and allow a feeling of peace within you,
refreshment. (*17*)
Be aware that all the time that tide of light has continued.
And as the light continues
then so does that flow of water. (*18*)

The counting technique is reversed here. Again it is used to give some structure to the process and emphasize a return to the initial levels of consciousness and attention. Instead of inducing sensations of quietness and stillness the emphasis changes to that of refreshment, joy and restoration. I stress this here because all too often we see meditation in a restricted way as inducing stillness and quietness, whereas at times we can use it to prepare for action or to be refreshed. All through the process I have been using the notion of flow in terms of light or of water. From the last line of the previous section I lead in to the next healing metaphor as illustrated below.

There was a fish, (*19*)
who somehow heard the word, Ocean.
And the fish asked 'What is Ocean, where is Ocean?'
No one knew.
The fish swam and searched and asked 'What is Ocean? Where is Ocean?'
and no one knew.
The fish searched and swam farther and farther, still asking the same question, 'What is Ocean, where is Ocean?'
Until, one day, the fish came to the place where the wise old fish lived and asked
'What is Ocean?' Where is Ocean?'
The wise old fish consulted.
'We have heard of this Ocean but we do not know Ocean.'
Eventually the fish died and disappeared.
The fish swam in Ocean, bred in Ocean, breathed in Ocean, lived in Ocean, was sustained by Ocean, reared its family in Ocean, was composed of Ocean, died in Ocean and became at one with Ocean.
We are the fish, God is the Ocean, (*20*)
Allow yourselves to arouse,
and to move and do whatever you wish to do
in your own time.
To move as you wish and to become aware of the others around you.
Allow yourself to recall whatever experiences you wish,

allow yourself the privacy of those experiences.
There is a time to talk
and a time to remain silent.
Amen.

I avoid any discussion of personal experiences immediately after a meditation. One of the reasons for this is that I want people to enjoy their understandings without putting a rational, linguistic overlay on them. Love, compassion, joy and healing are experienced profoundly within our hearts and are always poorly represented by words.

Another reason is that I am not concerned so much with what people say they have learned from the meditation, but with what then happens in their daily lives. The fruits of this way of working should be readily discernible by the persons themselves, by those with whom they live and by their friends. A by-product of working in this way is that in personally experiencing peace at a number of levels, i.e. physical, psychological, spiritual, and social, then we begin to recognize both unrest and peace within others. Again I urge you to try the experiment of fostering calm deep within yourself and seeing what effect this has on others. This week calm, next week love perhaps?

Children respond to this way of working very readily. They seem far more willing to exercise their imaginations than do we fossilized adults. In a local school young people were keen to try this out and entered into the process with great enthusiasm. I wonder what would be the result in terms of health if we practised in this way each day with our own children.

In our youth confirmation group I led brief meditations lasting for two minutes at a time and counting from 5 down to 1. The children aged between 11 and 16 enjoyed these brief moments of quiet. It also introduced them to a spiritual discipline which they could use within their own lives.

By far the most extensive use I have made of these techniques is for clinical problems.

First, I use the audiotape of the first session to introduce people to my voice and give them a chance to see whether or not they want to try the method. The ability to turn a tape on or off gives the listener complete control.

Second, I make a home visit and we discuss the area to be healed. I will then record a new tape, with the person, of a meditation constructed especially for them. To do this I use a portable cassette tape recorder and lapel microphone. This recording need not take place in the home – I have made recordings in the hospital ward at times when pain relief has been crucial. Most often the tape allows a time of rest and is a precursor to sleep which can occur quite spontaneously.

Apart from the physical benefits of meditation I concentrate on mobilizing the personal and spiritual resources of the person. Many people who suffer chronic pain or have a life-threatening illness not only need solace and comfort but are fearful for the future, and are concerned that their will to keep on living is being eroded. I will then construct a meditation based on these concerns. By the skilful use of Bible stories it is possible to transport the person to a place distant in time. By elaborating their perceptions of smell, touch, hearing and sight they can sit at the feet of Christ and hear what he has to say to them. For some people I ask them to sit on a hillside and hear what Christ has to say about the meek, and the poor. For others I take them to a distant shore by a lake and ask them to set out in a boat. On the water, at a time of peace in the light of a fading day, they can encounter Christ who will talk to them and touch them.

Not all meditation has to be done with our eyes closed. We can become quiet and then open our eyes. Seeing the natural world from a state of peace can be a revelation. The hand of God appears in all that exists. This can be tried quite simply.

Sit in front of a vase of flowers. Close your eyes. Count down from 5 to 1, all the time being filled with light. Then, open your eyes and simply see.

The same can be done with music, but allowing oneself to hear. I do this before reading a passage from the Scriptures as an aid to learning. All too often I jump to old conclusions. By becoming still I can be open to learning, open to the Word, open to becoming 'en*light*ened'.

I hope you have some idea now of how to proceed. Use this meditation if you wish. Invariably it will change as you adapt it to meet the needs of those you are with. Prayers can be inserted at different places. This helps people to assimilate the process by giving them something with which they are conversant. Invite others to join the group and ask them to rewrite the meditation using a particular biblical passage or the readings for that week. By introducing meditation to the home groups then I have given members of our parish the opportunity to try something new. It is from these meditations that the word has gone out about meditation. This has led to people in distress requesting help. One person tells another. I do not have to convince people. They request this help. These requests come through personal contact of friends and acquaintances. In this way our health becomes a communal endeavour and we all share in collective resources.

4 *Healing Services*

In our parish, it has been through the formal healing services that many people have been introduced to the laying on of hands for healing. Within the tradition of the Church as a whole the sacrament of laying on of hands has been used as a means of commissioning people for service, and as a sign of adoption within the community of believers. Healing services fulfil an important function within the life of the Church. Not only do they provide ministry to individuals, but are a means of building up the whole body of the Church.

Within our church the healing services have been seen as a part of the whole of communal church life. We have been wary of separating 'healing' into some precious category removed from all the other activities going on within the church. My perspective is that it is the whole active process of the Christian life which brings healing. The formal, sacramental activity is only a part. Without love there is no healing. However, it is a vital and necessary part which meets many people at their point of need.

Similarly, in the context of a healing service, the laying on of hands is part of the whole. It would be wrong, I believe, to say that healing only occurs during the laying on of hands. The whole service is important. The praise, the confession, the absolution, the Word, the intercessions and that ultimate sacrament of healing, the Eucharist, are all vital components. Rather than separate out bits and pieces we can begin to appreciate 'wholes', and to understand where one part informs another. This is a metaphor of our life within the body of the Church. We all play important and vital parts together.

When we gather together then we present ourselves with the opportunity to love each other, and to share in a context where we are loved. Healing services are an opportunity to show that Jesus loves his followers. Rather than talk about the love of God we are given an opportunity to experience the love of God. Here, in a formal church service, we are offered an immediate expression of compassion. Not only are we given the chance to be reached out to and touched, but also the chance to learn how to accept compassion. It is possible for many of us to struggle through our lives, holding off others in our vain attempts to be self-sufficient. Healing is located in the relationships we have with other people. It is not a one-way activity; no matter what it is that we are offered we have to learn to accept that offer.

Within the healing service we can both 'reach out' and be 'reached'. The importance of the laying on of hands is the simplicity with which this message is conveyed. Reaching out, being touched, are real activities and outside the use of words. When a person comes forward for healing we see not only the offer of God's love symbolized by the hands reaching out, but the offer by the person coming forward to be touched, showing thereby that they are willing to accept that love, to be part of that loving and Divine relationship.

However, healing is not solely located in this act alone. Healing of the sick by prayer or the laying on of hands, or anointing with oil, is part of an activity which belongs to the whole community. As communities we must meet these challenges such that our 'health' is seen as an activity in which we all engage. Every act of love for a person who is sick is part of the sacrament. Every kindness to the person who is weary or heavy laden is a sacramental act which is part of the healing ministry. As communities we can reach out to those isolated within our midst whether by creed, ethnic origin or social status, and also to other communities. As Christians we cannot say that we are healed if the old die alone, if our children despair, if our neighbours are spurned for what they believe or for the colour of their skin or if there are those among us who are impoverished. We must be vigilant that we do not contribute to that impoverishment by neglect.

Healing cannot be limited to the activity of priest to penitent. Healing becomes an activity in which we all share. We are the body of Christ, and in the sharing of his love, by our reaching out to each other, then his body is in the world again. The challenge for us as individuals is to set apart our 'selves' and to love over and over again such that collectively we become all compassion, all that is love.

Setting up the healing service

From the beginning we decided at St George's, Wilton, that we would not advertise our healing services beyond the local parish. This was not a parochial desire to be exclusive and minister only to ourselves. Our intentions were to build up slowly within our own parish to meet local needs, and to learn as we went along. We knew what we must do but we had no depth of experience in terms of a 'healing' ministry to call upon.

Furthermore, we were concerned that our activities should not inhibit the work of others. Before we began our services I had been to other churches to see what they did during healing services and to look at what other 'healers' did. My concern from these visits was that people would come from far and wide to see particular healers and by doing so miss the opportunity to minister to each other within their own congregations. Certainly people came for healing and their individual needs were met, yet there was no broader understanding that healing is a corporate activity.

The gifts of the Spirit are for building up the body of the Church, and while individual healings are paramount, it is this corporate activity which must not be ignored.

The very first healing service did vary slightly from these intentions as Bishop Morris Maddocks and his wife, Anne, were able to come and talk to us in the afternoon before leading our service in the evening. To make the most of this visit we invited other local churches to come and hear what Bishop Morris had to say about healing, and then to stay on for the evening service. My lasting impression from this beginning was that so many people came from varying Christian traditions, and differing walks of life. Talking about healing brought us together as Christians.

It is this aspect of healing which I believe is so important in the wider community whereby the Church itself becomes healed. We are being offered an opportunity at this time in the twentieth century, when beset by so many problems and when words are used as weapons to promote division, to come together, to love each other, to forgive and be compassionate in a way which is not dependent upon words but upon the simple activity of reaching out.

The people involved in the laying on of hands at this first service were Bishop Morris Maddocks, our parish priest, a local general practitioner, and myself. This professional or male domination has now changed. We have a preponderance of lay persons as part of our group concerned with healing, and the majority of these are women. This change occurred because we believed that church leadership was again being firmly controlled by men and that the healing ministry as a 'new' endeavour within our church was a real opportunity to redress the balance and promote equality.

The structure of the service

The structure of our formal services has stayed very much the same, although we have experimented with informal approaches at other times. I will describe these later in the chapter. One of the reasons for maintaining a formal service was that visitors, or our own parishioners even, could feel at home with the service and need not feel exposed to anything strange. On reflection I think that we have erred on the side of caution. However, we have been continually careful of others. It is not just *our* Church, i.e. it does not belong to those who are vocal or innovatory, but to all the parishioners. I would have felt that we had failed if anyone was prevented from attending because of what we were doing.

Basically the service takes the form used for celebrating the sacrament of the Eucharist. So far this has always been at evensong, and even if there has been a celebration of the Eucharist earlier in the day. When there is no Eucharist celebrated then the form is still the same in the earlier parts of the service.

There are published services for the sick. A booklet called '*Ministry to the Sick*' *Authorized Healing Services* is available from the publishers of *The Alternative Service Book 1980*. This is written for the Church of

England. An ecumenical service is published by the Acorn Healing Trust and can be obtained from Whitehill Chase, Bordon, Hants.

The form we use is as follows:

The preparation

First, those who are involved in leading the service will get together and pray. This is not solely those who will lay on hands, but also the readers, and the group leading the singing and worship. The service will have been planned beforehand and this usually involves several people meeting together to co-ordinate activities, and to work around a general theme. For instance, if I were to give an address on the importance of forgiveness then I would ask those involved to prepare songs around forgiveness, and select various readings to demonstrate forgiveness. This planning is not meant to be rigid and exclude spontaneity, or omit any songs which depart from the theme. In some cases it is the departures which highlight the central theme.

The intention is to place a particular thematic emphasis running like a thread throughout the service which people can discern as being woven through the fabric of their own lives. In this way we teach others and learn ourselves at a number of differing levels, through a number of channels as I emphasized in the last chapter. Some of us 'hear' through the words of the readings or the address. Others 'hear' in the music. Others may 'hear' in the broader rhythms of the service as it unfolds for them emotionally and spiritually.

For many it is in the touch where their needs are met. I like to believe that it is in the whole atmosphere of love reflected in the words and music which prepares the environment for healing to take place, in the way in which a gardener prepares the soil

Welcome. When people come into the church they are welcomed informally by a sidesperson, and sometimes by one person going over to say 'hello'. I have always believed that when people step into the church building they should be offered some expression of welcome. I know this can fall into an effusive assault which may impinge on the reverence of some parishioners and this is to be guarded against. However, in the celebration of healing then a spoken kindness, or a simple handshake can convey acceptance, welcome and a willingness to share. The gentleness of touch, no matter how brief, is a powerful indicator of shared humanity.

If we consider that some people who ask for healing can rarely articulate their problems, or the depth of their hurt, then reaching out to touch them is fundamental. It conveys both acceptance and the notion that there is no necessity to get tangled up in words. We become so tangled up in spoken language (yes, and written!), that we forget the importance of touch. For the lonely, for those who are in pain, for those with a life-threatening illness, or those who feel deep shame, human contact is the first step in feeling that they are being reached out to. To become one body we have to reach out and join with others. For those who feel abandoned we have to reach out and embrace them.

Hymn. Then we sing. Whether we use traditional hymns or modern songs it is important to unify ourselves in a common expressive activity. After this hymn the person responsible for the service will offer a short passage from the Bible pertinent to the service and say a few words of welcome. There is then a short period of silence and reflection. This is essentially a time of waiting to allow the 'busyness' of the day to be set to one side, to become quiet and prepare ourselves for an awareness of the presence of the Holy Spirit.

Prayer. Then follows a prayer. Although this is the place traditionally used for the prayer of penitence we usually move this to the alternative, later place within the Eucharist service. We use this as a time of giving thanks and worship in prayer. Tentatively at first, but with increasing confidence, we have encouraged those in the congregation to contribute spontaneously to this time of prayer. To help accomplish this the president of the service will say that anyone who feels they would like to say a one-line prayer of thanks for whatever has happened to them in their recent daily life may do so. The president begins this session of prayer, and brings it to a close. I use the term 'president' as this part of the service is usually organized by one particular person, who does not have to be a member of the clergy.

Praise and worship. We then have a period of praise and worship in song. Many people are released emotionally, and touched spiritually by the use of music within the service. Music has been used throughout the ages both as a part of ritual and as an aid to spiritual awareness. Paradoxically, while for some people the lyrics are important in sacred songs, for others it is the very non-verbal nature of music which is the most important factor. However, it is in praise that we give glory to God and we can all do that no matter how well or ill we feel, or whatever our state of grace. Furthermore, Jesus exhorts us to give glory so that we may be united in the Father. In the singing of our common song then we become one. Perhaps when we sing a greater common song outside the Church then our unity will become apparent to all.

It is also in this unity that we can experience understandings of the nature of healing. By giving praise we can 'give'. No matter how wretched we feel, we can still praise, or be part of 'praising' in the company of others. It is a release from a self-focused existence to an 'other'-focused existence. We move outside ourselves and our temporal concerns to a greater understanding of a spiritual reality which we share.

At a psychological level we are given the opportunity to break up regular patterns of specific behaviour where our thoughts follow repetitive patterns and we become open to broader holistic understandings.

Instead of falling back into patterns of thought which may be unfulfilling or return us to our worries, we can break out and be released to the fullness of the world and all our inherent potential. A feature of depression appears to be the continuing repetition of self-defeating patterns of thought which construe any event as negative and lead the sufferer into a lifestyle where nothing new is ventured, because the outcome is always failure or disappointment. Praise in the form of singing can break up these patterns.

At the simplest of physical levels, while singing we are breathing in a different way. The very activity of breathing differently using both our full lung capacity and our diaphragm is in itself beneficial. It is this very activity which is being taught as an aid to relaxation, as a part of meditation, and which I use for teaching others as part of a self-care package. In singing, as a form of praise and worship, we have the best of both worlds and a 'naturalistic' activity with which some people are more comfortable than with particular breathing techniques.

The word

In our service we choose the readings carefully to complement the address. After the first reading we will sing an appropriate hymn, or our singing group will either teach us a new song or sing to us. In the tradition of sacred music, songs have been used to lead the listener to a state of receptivity as well as to praise God.

In our church we like to take the opportunity to sing to others. By singing we can minister to them in a way which touches them deeply. Listening is not passive. We have to become receptive, and in this developing receptivity, at this time of being sung to, then we prepare the ground for healing. Being sung to can be disturbing for some people. I don't mean because the singing is unmusical, rather that they are moved deeply within themselves. This emotional release may move them to tears, and threaten the front with which they face the world. Sometimes people can be fearful that once they begin crying they will not stop.

It is important that, if people do appear to be distraught, they are offered some support after the service. However, weeping is nothing to be ashamed of. Sometimes in the process of our healing we need to experience release. If people do cry, do not immediately leap to the conclusion that they are distressed. There are such things as tears of joy!

There will then be another reading which leads to the address or sermon. We have varied in our approach to the sermon. Sometimes we use this time for teaching directly about healing and wholeness, using the scriptural readings as a basis. At other times we invite people to come and talk about their work as Christians in healing, either as part of their work, or as a particular ministry. The previous scriptural readings will tie in with what they have to say.

Occasionally people will speak about their own healing experiences as a personal witness. Two general practitioners who are colleagues of mine have taken this opportunity to speak about their work from the basis of their own healing. Incidentally, both of these practitioners are women. It does seem to me to be a common experience, as I visit many healing centres, that women are far less inhibited than men in talking about their own vulnerability, and are more willing to submit themselves to being healed spiritually. Perhaps it is a recognition on their parts of the interconnectedness between their bodies, their emotions and their life-style.

This witness is all the more impressive for being delivered by qualified medical practitioners: not because being a doctor gives them any monopoly on truths about healing, but because they can speak of the interplay between orthodox medicine and spiritual healing. For a mother to talk about the marvel of a seriously sick child being treated with the best of modern pharmacology, and with the greatest of medical skill (from a background where she herself has received her training and employment), yet supported by prayer, meant that there was a recognition of all the healing gifts working together. Here indeed was an expression of wholeness where all aspects of existence were assimilated. Neither was denied, and each was celebrated.

Similarly for a successful colleague to talk about the difficulties of depression, the feelings of failure that this brought in her marriage and the guilt this provoked in her relationship with her children, taught us all many things about how weakness can become transformed into strength. Instead of being hidden and denied her vulnerability became the very platform on which she was able to reach out to others. This too is where healing lies. Not in the cure, but in the transformation.

I am sure that her success within the Church and within medicine is based upon that transformation, and upon her willingness to submit to the power of the Holy Spirit within her and the humility to be transformed by the Spirit.

At the end of the address an announcement is made before the service continues. The president will announce that the following sequence will involve prayers and the laying on of hands. Everyone present is invited to come forward for healing if they wish. They can also come forward to receive healing for someone else. In this way it is possible for friends and relatives to come forward for healing for those who are absent or distant. Those who do not feel they can come forward publicly are reassured that the whole service is concerned with healing and that not coming forward does not exclude them from being healed.

The congregation are also told that, when they go forward to receive the laying on of hands, they can, if they wish, tell the person who is to lay on hands what their problem is. For those who do not wish to do this, or who cannot articulate their problem it is sufficient to hold whatever their problem is, or for whomsoever they pray, in their heart.

Intercession

After the sermon or address we begin a series of prayers. The way we structure this is to ask one person to take charge of the prayers. He or she will be part of the team involved in the healing ministry and will have been party to the planning. The theme running through the readings and the address will be incorporated in these prayers.

We then use the prayer of penitence immediately before the laying on of hands. Forgiveness, I believe, is such a central activity for healing. Not only the desire to ask for forgiveness, but also the ability to accept that forgiveness. In my work with marital problems it is the two poles of forgiving which are important. One pole is a partner truly asking forgiveness and, incidentally, recognizing there is something to forgive. The other is for a partner to accept forgiveness graciously and not continue a cycle of resentment. Forgiving is an act of relationship: both participants have to be involved.

Those involved with the laying on of hands go forward first to the altar rail and pray for each other in pairs. Each partner lays on hands in turn. They then face the congregation from behind the rail, and those to receive the laying on of hands come forward.

We lay on hands in pairs. One person lays on hands directly, and the partner puts one hand on the person to receive healing and the other on the person laying on hands. The person laying on hands prays spontaneously. Although we begin our healing services with individuals laying on hands we moved to couples for two reasons. One was the simple expedient of introducing new members of the healing ministry to the experience of laying on hands in a service with an experienced partner. The second was that in our ministry we minister to others in pairs and this seemed a valuable opportunity to reinforce that approach.

Within our growing team there has been a shift from professional people to those from a wide variety of career and educational backgrounds. Their incorporation within the service has also been a public validation of the part they are to play within the ministry.

When the person to receive healing comes forward they usually tell the person who is to lay on hands what they wish healing for, although this is not absolutely necessary. It does appear to be important for some of those who come forward to be able to say what they wish to be healed, amost as if the very statement of the problem itself brings a freedom from it. For my own part I think we make far too much of what we say and of what people say to us, and that the laying on of hands is sufficient. It is God's grace which is freely given, and which does not need our continual chattering. The people come forward as a file and go to the couples who are available. They then return to their seats. We have a singing group who will sing a selection of songs at this time. The congregation are given the numbers of these songs so that they may join in if they wish.

We do offer counselling to people when necessary, either before or after the service, to give them a chance to talk about their problems, although I have resisted this for several reasons. First, it seems an unnecessary prolongation of what is already a long service. Second, I am sceptical about the nature and quality of what purports to be Christian counselling; we do not always have the resources of time or trained personnel within our parish. Third, it is God who heals. Talking about some things over and over again only interferes with that process. Finally, I have found that the desire to counsel in some people reflects their desire to be needed and does not always meet the need of the person to be counselled. We have a network of support which I will describe later, and there is a need for Christian counselling, but not always as part of the healing service.

The ministry of the sacrament

We share the peace together. As in many churches this is a time of great activity with a lot of hugging and kissing. Fortunately I enjoy and get a lot of hugs and kisses but I do worry that it can become rather concentrated among the 'in' crowd, and exclude others.

Sharing the peace is vital to our faith, and needs to be active, but we must be vigilant about only sharing the peace with those whom we know or feel peaceful towards. Going out to others is risky but we are encouraged to do this in the Gospels. All we are asked to do is say 'Peace be with you'. It is up to the other person to return that peace. Perhaps we all need to be aware that we are responsible for offering the peace in a manner which is acceptable to the other person.

We then continue with the eucharistic prayers and the administration of the sacraments.

The service finishes with a hymn and the dismissal. We do offer coffee afterwards in the church as an opportunity for people in the congregation to talk together with their friends or to contact members of the healing ministry. It is often at this time when we hear of others who wish to be prayed for or visited.

The structure of the service reflects that of the sacrament of the Eucharist as found in the Alternative Service Book of the Church of England, and is as follows:

The Preparation	hymn
	welcome
	prayer
	a time of praise and worship

Ministry of the Word	reading
	hymn
	reading
	sermon or address
Intercession	prayer
	confession/prayer of penitence
	laying on of hands
Ministry of the Sacrament	the peace
	preparation of the gifts
	eucharistic prayer
	administration of the sacraments
	hymn
	dismissal

Informal services

While the majority of our healing services have taken this formal approach and occupy a central sacramental role in our healing ministry we have experimented with a different approach. In visiting other churches outside the Church of England which have freer forms of expression, I have found that healing as an activity, and the laying on of hands in particular, appear to be more readily acceptable within the context of worship.

In some churches there seems to be some hesitation about recognizing the particular gift of healing as resident within one particular individual, and more of an expectation that if one person is in need then a fellow Christian will reach out a hand and heal, trusting in the Spirit. In this approach less emphasis is placed on the person as a healer, and more emphasis is placed on the healing community. Such expressions appear to be cultural, in that within particular sects there will be varying forms of expression, and these will be validated according to the traditions and practices of that sect.

Within our church we have a broad spread of ages and beliefs. Some people want a regular standard orthodox approach which gives them some measure of stability in a changing world. Our formal service appears to satisfy this need. Others, however, demand a freer form of expression which to them is more intimate and meets their need. I say 'to them' deliberately, as it is in formality and order that some people feel closer to God. In the absence of a personal involvement there is 'less of them' and 'more of God'.

I appreciate this view. In some services it can appear that each person or group is out to be more spirit filled or gifted than the next, rising on a crescendo of emotion which has little to do with the Holy Spirit and more to do with human sentiment. Yet it is a personal involvement with God which people want, and for some the presence of the Holy Spirit is an emotional experience. My concern is that some people never take up the challenge and go beyond the ecstasy. I think that this is, in part, caused by the way in which some religious experiences are structured in relation to the service. Some services follow the same format where people are encouraged through song, prayer and ritual to reach a certain state of spiritual ecstasy. However, while this is necessary in terms of evangelism and necessary for many of us (me included) as a 'real' celebration of the Spirit at work within us, I do believe it is limiting.

We need to understand and recognize the Holy Spirit at work in other areas of our life. It may not be that we are 'spirit filled' only in celebration, but that we are 'spirit filled' all the time. It could well be that it is only in celebration that we recognize the Holy Spirit within us. The task we must set ourselves is to forget our 'selves' in other contexts, or conversely to recognize the Holy Spirit at work within us at all times and in all places.

To try out healing in a different format we used the venue of a mid-week service which was lay led and informal. We met in an upper room of the church hall.

The service began with singing. Some of the songs were planned, and some were in response to requests from those present. We then had a period of praise where we thanked God for what he had done for us, or for our friends and families. We sang again and the songs were interspersed with readings which had been chosen by some of the people present.

This led into a meditation. I lit a candle in the room and led those present on a guided meditation on 'light' (see Chapter 3). The people present were asked to look at the candle and then to close their eyes and visualize the candle flame continuing to burn. The rest of the meditation continued on the theme of the light within us, and the light outside us gradually becoming one light until we, and those with us, became filled with the light of Christ.

We sang again. This was not solely to indulge my desire to sing. It is important to move between passivity and activity, from listening to expressing. When people are allowed to sing they can feel that they are an active part of the service. This is evident too in the expectation that people will take part in a time of praise and spontaneous prayer. I don't mean that in the sense of 'You will now all be spontaneous and pray'. Rather that an atmosphere is invoked whereby all present are encouraged to recognize that they have a voice to use, and something valuable to contribute.

By distracting from one activity, i.e. meditation, to another activity, singing, then the experience of meditating is allowed to become part of the person at a 'deep' level of consciousness and is not mediated by immediate thoughts. By singing, the people involved are not given the opportunity to make the usual sense of what has happened to them by putting verbal labels on their inner processes, but those processes are allowed to work within them uncluttered, or uninterrupted by verbal labels.

A time of teaching followed the meditation. The first part involved a reflection on the biblical precedent for healing as presented in the Gospels using the gospel stories. My main argument was that all too often we get caught up in the mechanics of healing (whether to lay on hands, use spittle and mud applied to the eyes, faith alone, prayer at a distance) when it is the activity of love which is the central concern, and focusing on Christ the Healer which is the paramount activity. When we love deeply then the mechanical actions fade into insignificance.

We then prayed for our hearts to be opened and that we would recognize Christ as he came to us. A song followed the prayer.

The next part of the teaching session involved each person reaching out to touch the person on their right-hand side and then on their left. This was accomplished with consummate ease. Each person was then asked to close their eyes and think of the person on their left, and then their right sitting in the light of Christ. A simple prayer was offered. Again a song followed this activity.

The main group was then divided into groups of three. These small groups were then asked to tell each other what they wished to pray for, and then to reach out to touch each other and pray for that person. And they did. There was no stopping them. The doubts some of us had about the participation of the group were dispelled. All around us people were talking together and reaching out to each other as if they did it all the time. What seemed, in the setting of the church, a formal and precious act, in another setting seemed quite as precious but very natural. There was no hesitancy and the questions were not about 'Have I the gift?', but 'Was there enough time to continue to meet all the needs?'

This informal healing has been replicated in the home groups mentioned in an earlier chapter. Given the opportunity, people welcome the chance to listen, to pray, to touch and to heal. Questions about how to lay on hands, where to put those hands, what to say and whether we have been ordained fade into insignificance. In terms of a living faith people act. Compassion is an activity, and is waiting to be released within each one of us.

We seem as a society to make the spiritual too far removed and distant from our everyday experiences. Spiritual concerns become accessible only to a few enlightened or called people. Our education system militates against the development and use of spiritual language such that spiritual understandings even when encountered cannot be built upon or articulated. This is a poverty which has far-reaching consequences. Not only are people starved and deprived now of these understandings which would feed their very being, but future generations are faced with a cultural desert and a spiritual famine. Christianity is a faith alive at the workbench, in the office, in the home and in the classroom. It is not reserved for mystics, seers and visionaries but is available for you and me. Our responsibility is to live our lives in the knowledge of a risen Christ. Reaching out to heal is one way of celebrating this knowledge.

5 Healing in the Home

There are times when we need individual attention. When we are feeling particularly vulnerable, we need to be cherished and listened to carefully. To meet this need we have developed our home-visiting activities. These can be separated into the visits made by people who belong to the team committed to praying with the sick and laying on hands and another group of people concerned with home visiting to the elderly housebound and the bereaved. This latter group falls more into the category of pastoral care, yet I would count all of these activities as part of the healing ministry.

Of course the parish priest has traditionally carried out the duty of visiting the sick and the bereaved as part of his pastoral role. However, at a time when there are fewer priests and ever-increasing demands on those priests in full-time ministry, it is not always possible to meet all the demands for visiting the sick or needy. Similarly, priests also recognize that their training does not meet all the counselling needs which they face in daily parish life. The pastoral role is not always a priority at theological college either for the priest or for the staff.

In our parish we began a series of joint home visits to people who asked for healing. These visits were predominantly instigated through the parish priest, but as we build up a network of support in the parish they are being instigated increasingly by other members of the healing ministry. The priest is always aware of who is being visited, and by whom. It is important to build up this network of shared information and to have someone who has an overall picture of what is going on. By doing so it is possible to avoid confusion, and to ensure that well-meaning attempts on the behalf of an individual do not interfere with what someone else is doing. There is nothing more galling than carefully to negotiate with a person, and their general practitioner, a way forward out of a difficult situation, then to find another person offering contradictory and confusing advice with only a partial understanding of the problem. This is not meant to prevent others being involved, rather to make sure that they are involved in a manner which uses their abilities wisely to assist the person who is to be helped.

These home visits are for the celebration of the Eucharist, for counselling, for the laying on of hands and to pray for, or with, the person. When a person is visited for the laying on of hands, or for prayer, then they are asked if they wish to invite other family members or friends along. These invitations are solely in their hands. Invariably in ministering to one person, another is helped. When one person suffers they rarely suffer alone. There are exceptions where true isolates exist, but our work is predominantly with people who have some social contact, either fraternal or familial.

In writing this I am struck by the fact that all too often our responses are made at times of difficulty, and our healing prayers and visits are seldom made in times of health. It could well be that we have this out of balance. Perhaps a next step is to celebrate in the home and to partake of healing in 'health' as well as 'sickness'.

Priest and counsellor

Our visits together follow a similar pattern. The people involved (priest and counsellor, priest and member of the healing ministry) arrange to meet at a person's house. The person is asked before by the priest if a colleague may attend with him. In a way this is an 'appointment' system and has to be so for several people to co-ordinate their different working lives. I have always tried to make it such that if one of the visitors has to leave for another appointment, the other person can remain. Having time for another person is in itself a healing activity. If one has to leave promptly, or for another appointment, one person will endeavour to spend some time socially in the home.

Initially some people were reluctant to have a person other than their priest to visit them. Then they were reluctant to have anyone other than the priest or myself. This reluctance has gradually been eroded as healing has been discussed within the parish and now a number of people are recognized as belonging to the healing team. As I have said before, the continual emphasis has been to move away from the individual 'body' to the notion of a healing community, the 'many as one body'.

The first part of the visit is spent in focusing on the problem and what the person is doing, or has done, to alleviate that problem. Many of the problems we encounter when we visit people have proved to be intractable to modern medical techniques.

In a way we have to understand not only the problem itself, but also the previous history which the person has gone through in attempting to solve their problem. Occasionally, before we even attempt to handle the problem itself we have to deal with feelings of failure about not recovering, resentment towards previous healing initiatives or, as I mentioned earlier, the confusion of conflicting advice from other persons involved with helping. Forgiveness itself is an essential part of healing.

Questions for the first visit

(1) Social questions

Who is living here with you?
Do you have many friends to visit?
Do they visit as often as you would like them to?

Do you see your family often? Where are they living?

These questions, apart from being incredibly nosy, help to build up a picture of whether the person is supported by a network of social contacts or is effectively isolated. (I will return to this in the next chapter when I write about helping families with cancer.) Furthermore, they give the person an opportunity to talk about their important relationships, and for you to discover any areas of interpersonal conflict.

(2) What is the problem?

Ask what the problem is exactly, and find out in clear terms how the person sees the problem. What you will need to know is when it occurs, and what happens. By doing this it is possible to pray specifically, and perhaps most importantly, to discern any changes. The more we identify particular problems then the easier it is to recognize change. I must emphasize that it is most important here to listen to what the person describes as the problem, and not to substitute your version of the problem. What I do is to make a clear statement back to the person of what I believe I have heard them say to me, in their words, and as exactly as possible. This is an act of love. By carefully listening to a person, to what they are saying exactly, and with total acceptance, we demonstrate a willingness to take their part. This does not mean that we have to abdicate our own views, rather that we open ourselves to others.

(3) What is a typical example of the problem?

Ask the person, or those present, to describe a typical example of the problem. You will need to find out who is present at the time the problem occurs, and where and when the problem occurs. If you find that someone is in pain, but that pain always occurs after a telephone call from an estranged family member, then it will be important to pray both for the relief of the pain *and* for the relationship between the person and the estranged relative.

(4) What changes do you expect?

It is important to identify the smallest possible changes. In this way the person begins to anticipate a healed future. I ask people the question 'if I came to your house again in three months time and sat with you here on your sofa what would you say had changed?' This immediately throws the person into a projected state where they are contemplating a future which includes a change in their circumstances. Rarely have I found that the person anticipates a worsening future.

When there is persistent and chronic pain, or a problem that has been present for a long time, I ask the person to rate their problem on a scale of 1 to 10, and then ask them what sort of reduction they expect. Sometimes this will be expressed as a percentage, i.e. 30 per cent reduction in pain. Sometimes as a number, i.e. the pain will fall from level 9 to a level of 6. Once again this gives us something specific to ask for in prayer. I am not discounting broad and general prayers, they are important. However, I do believe that specific prayers are answered and we can be encouraged to pray in this way. These changes may appear to be quite modest, but are what the person asks for. Trust them to ask for what is most appropriate. Yet again the healing for some people is to be listened to carefully, and recognized for their own competence. What a tragedy if a person asked for a 20 per cent reduction and were castigated by a counsellor for asking for too little! Should they ask for only 20 per cent and find total relief then all to the good. No matter how skilled or experienced we become we never have the gift of immaculate perception. Accept the other person, listen to their needs.

(5) What other methods have you tried to solve the problem?

I like to know what else the person has tried simply to avoid going around in circles and trying to repeat old, and failed solutions. Similarly if a person has exhausted a number of trained and skilful counsellors I will steer clear of any counselling endeavours. It is at these times when people can, if appropriate, talk about the difficulties they have had with other practitioners or with the frustration of the hospital appointment system. This is a further area which can be prayed about, and it is also possible to devise practical strategies for information-gathering. I spend time with people who are experiencing difficulties with their doctors: in working out exactly what they want to know, exactly what questions they have to ask and from whom they can find out the answers. Writing questions down on paper and taking this paper to the next consultation helps people steer a path through the confusion of sometimes conflicting advice and often an overload of information. When we hear information or advice at times of great stress it is all too easy to perceive wrongly what we are told. By having some guidelines and planning the consultation it is possible to separate fact from supposition.

Sometimes it is important simply to give detailed advice. I recently saw a man and his wife and could give them advice about sickness benefit and the supplementary benefit claims procedure. Not very spiritual you may say, but it brought much relief. Perhaps we have to beware of limiting healing to the few ways in which we see it and learn to look for healing in all activities.

The general practitioner

My own view is that the general practitioner is always the primary health-care agent for the family and that it is misguided to initiate any activities without involving him or at least gaining his compliance.

Before offering the person any direct help I always get them to contact their doctor and ask if I may be involved. Sometimes I will ask the general practitioner myself, but predominantly it is the responsibility of the person to ask their doctor. By working in a community over a period of time this is a welcome opportunity for co-operation between Church and medicine. It is not easy, but mistrust and misunderstandings can be dissolved with tolerance and openness on both sides.

Of course the parish priest does not have to acknowledge this courtesy. But, I do believe that our communal health concerns need the active co-operation between clergy and medicine. By a willingness to inform each other the first steps to heal the relationship between the two can be made. If regular meetings between a local health centre and the clergy/healing team could be made there would be real opportunities for healing endeavours in their broadest sense. If the sacraments could be celebrated in a health centre once a month then another move could be made which would shift the stereotypes of particular health activities away from their specific locations of surgeries or churches. Ideally relationships with the local health centre should begin as soon as you are considering your healing ministry. Most general practitioners are willing to listen. One way is to tell them what you try to do to keep yourself healthy, or how you overcome your problems using prayer, with the help of a Christian counsellor or through a healing sacrament. Be bold, lovingly.

The format for home visits

Feeling at ease

The first part of the visit is spent in helping the person to feel at ease. An advantage of being in the person's home rather than in a clinic or the vicar's study is that the person is already on their own territory and in control of the situation. While I generally insist on seeing people for counselling or therapy outside of their home, the reverse is true for the laying on of hands.

Inevitably we will be offered a cup of tea or coffee. I invariably accept. This allows the person to do something for you. It is a useful social activity to begin a relationship which may initially feel awkward for all parties involved. First, it gets away from the expectation that what is about to happen is necessarily a solemn and formal affair. Second, it allows the person to do something while they talk. Third, it often gives you a chance to talk in the informal surroundings of the kitchen rather than the formality of another room. My own theory is that, when I have graduated to the position of being shown immediately into the kitchen, then I have been accepted by the person and their family.

Talk over the problem

We then talk over the problem and the previously attempted solutions as mentioned earlier. This is the time to discover from the person what they expect, and to ask them why they have asked us to visit. This may have already been discovered by the parish priest but I like to hear it first hand. Sometimes people have had time to think and have become clearer in their ideas. This is done with those present sitting in their easy chairs, or on the floor in some houses if people are particularly relaxed or there are several friends present. Occasionally when other people are present the problem may change slightly, or those others present may ask for something for themselves. For example, the spouses of people we see often ask for peace of mind, or patience, or prayers of comfort too. This is also a good time to find out the views of those present about Christian healing.

Say what is to be done

The next stage is to tell the person what we will do and to give our perspective on healing. We tell them that there will be a reading, followed by a time of prayer and then we lay on hands together (and sometimes anoint with oil).

Our expectation is that they will be expectant. Healing will occur but the onus is on us all to recognize that healing. Sometimes people feel better immediately, there is relief from anxiety and a sense of being accepted and loved. At a later date some people find that there is a physical change which exhibits itself as a relief from symptoms, or shows itself as a physical change when viewed on being X-rayed. For some people the change comes in terms of accepting circumstances and a new approach to life. For others there is a change in relationship with those they love, or live with. Yet others experience a change in their spiritual understandings, they may become freer, or more alive or understand that they are forgiven. The importance of setting the minimum expectations which I mentioned earlier is that people know when their prayers are answered, and when they are answered in abundance they are even more aware of the gift.

Whatever happens, our duty is to stand back and wait, and to marvel. While there are reports of immediate and spectacular cures these have not been my experience. I am wary of cheap grace, as if all we have to do is to go into a situation, lay our hands on the sick, and see them miraculously cured like some psychic magicians. What we are all a part of, and what we occasionally catch a glimpse of, is the process which Hans Küng describes, of 'all creation being healed'. To accomplish this each person must play their part. The healing is in each person being involved with another, not in the materialism of cure. It is love which is the sign which transforms suffering to salvation. In this way we see people living in the same circumstances yet experiencing them differently. It is possible to say that, on the one hand, sometimes nothing changes, but, on the other hand, everything changes.

Of course there are changes which defy scientific logic. I would not be part of this ministry if I had not seen reversals in the progress of an invasive cancer, changes in skin conditions, movement from depression to joy, and the healing of relationships. But what I have seen, which is greater than these 'miracles', is people committed to each other through long periods of struggle without giving up on each other, the love and constancy of nursing spouses through senile dementia, neighbours persevering in the face of rejection, and the compassion and caring of families at times of dying. If we miss these healings and the message that they have for the world then we are depriving our communities of the Christian message: 'Love heals'.

Forgiveness

We use the Alternative Service Book as the basis for our home healing if we are to lay on hands and anoint with oil, and particularly if we are to celebrate the Eucharist. We begin with the prayers of penitence. This part is read by the parish priest and the responses made by those present.

Reading

There then follows a reading. This is chosen as being pertinent to the particular problem of the person. This is easier if you know what the problem is before you call or have an extensive knowledge of Scripture. As I rarely know beforehand what the exact problem is, nor do I possess an elaborate knowledge of the Scriptures, I rely on a few readings which I find satisfying and which offer examples of God's promise to us. More often than not I use something from the Servant Songs in Isaiah or a direct reporting of what Christ said from the Gospels.

Intercessory prayer

We then pray together. Anyone present is asked to join in if they wish. One person takes responsibility for beginning and ending this time of prayer. Sometimes people wish to kneel at this time and I will join them, otherwise we remain seated. If we have visited often it is good to hear other people joining in with the prayers and praying for each other. It is at these times I do realize how much the Church is the people and not the stone buildings. To be in a friend's house with their neighbours or family, some of whom might be strangers to us, and hear them take the first tentative steps to active prayer is a marvellously invigorating and spiritual experience. The effect it has had for me is to make me less tentative in offering to pray with strangers. People have spiritual needs and prayer is the door which leads to those needs being met.

Laying on of hands and anointing with oil

Usually we lay on hands in pairs. I will lay both hands on the person who remains sitting or kneeling. My partner will put one hand on top of mine and the other hand on my arm or shoulder. In some ways this resembles a triangle of contact. I will then pray for that person, and ask God for what they have asked, in the words that they have said to me. If I feel intuitively that I need to place my hands on a place other than on their head then I will do so. The other person in the healing pair is also free to pray too.

My praying I must admit has become briefer and to the point. When I first started I prayed very elaborately as if I were being commissioned to compose a minor epic. The more I have been asked to pray and the more those prayers have been answered, then the more I have realized how little I need to do. So now I pray simply and reflect what the person asks for.

The laying on of hands does not have to be restricted to the priest or his partner. In a home Eucharist for a friend, one of his family friends was visiting from London before returning to Australia. She asked to lay on hands to pray for her friend. This was a beautiful and 'touching' occasion. The expression of love was a real indication of God's healing being present and available to all of us. For me it was an invaluable chance to sit on the sidelines and be free to observe one person ministering to another.

Sometimes we will anoint with oil. The oil is kept in the church and is taken from the oil which is blessed in the cathedral on Maundy Thursday. This anointing follows the laying on of hands and is usually done by one person only. As the oil is in a small bottle I put my thumb over the open end and tip the bottle upside down. Using my thumb I make a sign of the cross upon the forehead of the person and say a prayer.

For some people the anointing with oil carries some associations with the sacrament of anointing the sick before death. A man I saw recently (who was dying, incidentally) asked that I didn't anoint him in the presence of his family as they would fear that his death was imminent. How right he was. First, to ask for the anointing, which he said brought him great peace. Second, because he did die within a fortnight. He knew within himself what he needed, and was aware of his own death.

I use the oil as a sacrament of thanksgiving to God and as a commissioning of the person anointed to 'go forward' whether into life or death. The thanksgiving is that which is represented in the story of Jacob who in the morning after his vision anoints the stone to revitalize the indwelling God. The commissioning is a message to persevere, to go out into the world revitalized. Healing is not an activity which ceases. We have to go out into the world and continue that task of loving our neighbour, and our enemy. It is for this task of Christian loving that we need all our vitality and for which we need to be healed.

After the healing I stay and talk for a while. Sometimes people like to talk about their experiences of healing. Others change the subject entirely and talk about their immediate plans. More often than not the people present are very quiet, at rest and at peace. I then leave quietly. My only stipulation is that I will not become engaged immediately in another round of counselling. So far nobody has asked me to do so anyway.

If people want us to visit again we leave it with them to initiate the contact unless we have already set a fixed pattern.

Celebration of the Eucharist

For me this is the sacrament of healing. After we have laid on hands the priest involved will prepare the bread and the wine. He brings this in a small case and uses wafers and wine which have already been consecrated. It is possible to use bread and wine from the house but the service then takes longer. We return to the Alternative Service Book and work directly from that, and include the sharing of the peace.

My feelings about the sacraments of healing and the Eucharist are reflected in the following passage by Carl Jung:

> This rite of his sacrificial death is not a repetition of the historical event but the original, unique, and eternal act. The experience of the Mass is therefore a participation in the transcendence of life, which overcomes all bounds of time and space. It is a moment of eternity in time [J. Jacobi (ed.), *C. G. Jung, Psychological Reflections* (Routledge & Kegan Paul 1953), p. 364].

As I have said before, the service of healing in the home is for all involved. Those involved in the service bring their needs too. For some people who are not regular churchgoers this is a gentle opportunity to remind them of God's love.

My approach is a soft evangelism if you like. Apart from an abhorrence of the spiritual colonialism of some groups who attempt to crush my understandings with their own certainty, I believe that all we need to do is to 'offer' love to others. We simply reach out to others and show them how their hunger can be fed and satisfied. They will eat when they are ready, and in their own time as God's Spirit moves within them. Force feeding can cause all sorts of aversions. Similarly we all have different dietary requirements and to impose one diet on another is counter-productive.

Pastoral care team

At the same time that the healing ministry was developing we were also aware in the parish of the need for people to be visited in their homes. This was particularly for the elderly living alone, and also for those who had been recently bereaved. To meet these needs a team of volunteers was gathered together, each of whom would each take on a person, or persons, to visit regularly. Each volunteer could take on whatever level of commitment was necessary for that person according to the needs of the visitor and the visited. The original referrals came through the parish priest, but as the group developed, the pastoral visiting team referred by word of mouth. All parishes have grapevines. Once the team was set up and actively working then people got to know about it. There is no fixed template for the style of these visits, people are given the freedom to adapt to what is best.

The visiting team is co-ordinated by a lay person who makes the original visit and endeavours to match the person to be visited with the most appropriate visitor from the team. There are regular meetings too. What we have lacked is any formal counselling training for volunteers and that is currently being planned. In a way it has been for the best to have a lack of formal training in that people have been reluctant to run before they can walk. There is no harm in starting small. From our modest beginnings built on the foundation stone of willing service, trusting in the guidance of the spirit, we can all achieve wonderful things.

The prayer chain

The prayer chain is a group of people who have agreed to pray for others. If any person knows of anyone who has a problem or who wishes to be prayed for they telephone the next person on the list with a prayer request. The information passed on is the name of the person initiating the prayer, the name of the person to be prayed for (unless that person wishes to remain anonymous), and the nature of the prayer request. Once this person has prayed they then pass the request on to the next person in the chain. By doing this many people can be involved quickly in praying for one person or their family. Consequently people are not only actively engaged in a meaningful and purposeful prayer life, but also actively engaged in the compassionate care of others. An additional benefit is that we also see the concrete results of our prayers being fulfilled. A prayer chain does not have to be a chain of sorrows or despair. We can, and do, use the chain for messages of thanksgiving. This is a remarkably simple way of promoting parish prayer life between people who may be quite scattered geographically. My only fear has been about it developing into a grapevine of gossip, but this fear has been unfounded.

Many paths

There are many paths to healing. Within our parish lives we can promote initiatives which meet the needs of parishioners and utilize their many and varied gifts. This chapter has I hope demonstrated how various initiatives meet the need for healing. There is no one pattern which can be applied. There are ideas that can be copied. However, at the heart of our endeavours is a willingness to be guided and counselled by the Spirit. What I do know is that once we set out upon the spiritual journey, of which healing is one road, then Christ fulfils his promise to us. His message is that he is the Way. Trusting to that we are not for ever lost. The more this ministry goes forward the more I am asked to pray with people and to heal. People ask not from an understanding of what I do, but from an intuitive knowledge deep within their own hearts. In the next chapter I hope to show how the healing ministry within a church can be used as a platform within the broader context: that of the community. We are sent out not to minister to ourselves but to others. I do not mean that we should neglect our Christian brothers and sisters, it is they who love and support us, but we must strive not to be complacent and shun the 'outside' world. It is there where we learn Christian love.

6 *Healing and Dying*

This chapter focuses on the management of terminal illness in the context of the family and uses the varying initiatives from the previous chapters. Several important issues are raised. First is a consideration of who is thought to be a family member. Second is the consideration of critical junctures in the process of dying. Third is a discussion of the way in which community professionals can co-ordinate their practice.

A feature of working with the terminally ill is that for the individual there will be no symptomatic recovery. This is not undue pessimism on my part, or a lack of faith. All too often we equate healing with curing. Any of us who choose to work with the terminally ill will find that no matter how hard we pray, no matter how many skills we learn or how earnestly we believe, people die. This does not mean that no healing occurs. It is we who limit the notion of healing. When we work with families where a person is dying and see them grow closer to Christ, when we pray with families and see pain reduced and hope restored such that a family member is released then healing does occur. All this may appear counter to a 'signs and wonders' ministry which emphasizes curing. We can see signs and wonders; they are often expressed as fortitude, in tears and in cheerfulness. In working with the dying we are taught about life. At such times we are privileged to come close to a spiritual reality which is central to our faith.

Although no symptomatic change occurs, there are problems which have to be resolved and accommodated. The family have to adapt to the process of losing a loved one, and then life continuing without that person. Appreciating the involvement of the wider family network and the influence of health professionals developed by family therapists is important in understanding the management of terminal illness.

The overriding emphasis in this chapter is one of assisting families to use their own resources to accommodate change. However, they are helped in this by a network of community support.

The context of the practice

This work is carried out in my capacity as a pastoral counsellor working in the church community, although the work could be carried out by the parish priest or anyone engaged in a leadership role in the local community. The use of the term 'pastoral counsellor' is deliberate. With such a term there is no connotation of change. There is an implication of listening and caring without any overtones of social welfare.

By working for a church organization it may appear that the delivery of the service is restricted to predominantly middle-class families. In practice no such restrictions exist on the grounds of income or class status. There is no discrimination either on the grounds of religious faith, or lack of it. Furthermore the experience of pain and the process of dying seem to have scant regard for income, material wealth, social status or state of grace.

Referrals

The initial referrals are made by the parish priest who hears about family problems in the course of his daily work. As in most communities there is a lay network of information. He then asks the family if they wish to be visited by both him and me for a preliminary interview.

The service offered is a 'holistic' approach to the management of terminal illness with an emphasis on understanding family change. By 'holistic' I mean a stance which attempts to integrate the body, the mind and the spirit. The specific activities offered are: prayer, the administration of the sacraments in the home, family counselling, meditation and visualization, and formal and informal hypnosis for the management of pain. It is important to stress here that this service is not concerned necessarily with some of the faddish techniques associated with 'holistic' medicine but the underlying principles which respect the patients' capacity to be involved in their own healing processes. Furthermore, they are regarded as active partners in their own health care rather than passive recipients. This means a change in stance by the practitioner from that of 'expert' to 'guide'.

In the course of working with the patient and the family the principal practitioners involved are: the parish priest, the family doctor, the specialist hospital consultants and, in the case of leukaemia, the specialist nursing sister. Apart from these persons there are parishioners who offer a range of necessary support activities. The emphasis then is on the 'body' of the community, where constituent parts come together. The healing begins in this process of unity.

It is easy to get carried away with formulating and implementing therapeutic regimes and dismiss the very important activities of child-minding while parents are visiting hospital, taking a person shopping or relieving a spouse from being at home all day. Similarly there are formal social groups which the spouse of the patient can attend or can be invited to attend. The sacrament of the neighbourly visit can be all too easily ignored.

It is this level of support which proves to be beneficial in the support of bereaved families. The friendships made during the course of dying are themselves therapeutic and far more ecologically sound than the formalities of therapy. Also, the person who is dying gains some comfort that their spouse is actively making friends and planning for a future which does not include the patient.

In addition the lay support for the family means that there is an emotional tie with the family before the patient dies. In this way there is no need for bereavement counselling. The family and the lay support network understand the grief and share that grief. Informal friendships with the family made at the time the person is dying persist.

In this community approach the function of the author is to oversee and co-ordinate the principal practitioners and lay network. In some cases this proves difficult if the general practitioner wishes to retain full control. This has been overcome by initially acceding to the wishes of the general practitioner. However, once the family doctor is able to see the benefit of a co-ordinated approach, particularly when the family doctor has run out of alternative interventions, then co-operation is possible. The approach by the consultant oncologists at the general hospital with whom I have worked is that anything which contributes to the welfare of a patient who is suffering the trauma of radiotherapy and chemotherapy is to be welcomed.

A feature of our work as Christians is to promote unity. It would be a tragedy if we, in trying to work together, promoted discord. I do not underestimate the difficulty of this task. However, I do know that when people become comfortable, when they are freed from pain, when they express hope, then inter-disciplinary frictions disappear. A central feature of any healing ministry, as I have written earlier, is to begin dialogues. Some of us do this through teaching or research. Some priests, counsellors and doctors meet at practice lunchtimes on a regular social basis. Beginning courses together, or inviting doctors to act as advisers, all promote co-operative endeavour.

Family change and terminal illness

Coping with physical changes	*the anticipation of pain the management of pain the management of the physical sequelae of illness (nausea, incontinence) change in physical appearance the management of the physical sequelae of treatment
Coping with personal change	*loss of hope, fitness, identity anxiety and depression about future loss of role in family and in employment frustration and helplessness
Coping with family and marital changes	resolution of conflict change in parental roles anxiety about future welfare (financial and emotional) anticipated loss of family member

	handling hospital contacts and treatment
	planning the future
	social isolation
	changes in boundary, and the negotiation of dependence/independence
	the negotiation of marital and family distance
	saying 'goodbye', and talking about dying
	handling the personal and physical changes described above
Coping with spiritual changes	*feelings of loss, alienation and abandonment
	understanding suffering
	accepting dependency, handling anger and frustration
	forgiving others
	discovering peace
	discussing death
	grieving
	planning the funeral

*Note that all these changes have ramifications throughout the interconnected systems. All personal changes have implication for other family and community members.

First contact

The first contact, after referral, is at the patient's home. Even if the patient is in hospital and has given consent to be visited this initial contact is made with the patient's spouse in the home. The spouse is then asked for their consent to visit the patient. This is not a breach of confidentiality. All the people I have worked with so far have relished the idea of information being shared and that someone has bothered to include them in the decision-making. It is the very lack of co-ordination which causes so many problems and anguish for patients. While the patient may have the disease, their spouses also have to cope with that 'dis-ease'. They have to answer innumerable telephone calls with equanimity. They have to be calm and patient while answering questions to which they have limited information at a time when they are not feeling particularly calm or patient. Friends and relations call for news of the patient's progress, yet who stops to ask the spouse about their own coping? To involve the spouse is to recognize their place as central alongside the patient in the future management of the illness.

At this first meeting the foundations of the future contacts are made. Any interventions are made from a basis of shared information with both partners and are under the influence of the patient and the spouse. The reason for this is that families where terminal illness is present express a loss of control over the therapeutic endeavour, and the process of dying itself comes to be seen as beyond their control. This realization can be frightening. I know some people will say that dying certainly is out of their control; but the way that realization is achieved, in the context of lived faith or as a sudden pronouncement, makes all the difference. Our theological abstractions about life and death can seem quite fragile in the living reality of dying.

The process of therapeutic intervention, the management of information and social support is brought into the realm of family influence. In this way responsibilities are shared and the process of change becomes a co-operative endeavour. The practitioners involved act as guides and facilitators.

For these families the future is inevitable and immediate. There are overt and visible expected changes. The expected change cannot be averted, simply anticipated. While we may have our own views about the future and feel quite optimistic, or spiritually secure, or that the patient is unduly pessimistic, we must beware of imposing these views on those whom we see. Their reality is different from ours. Working with the dying raises all our own fears about our own mortality. It is all too easy to offer a counsel of optimism or spiritual platitudes to protect our own understandings rather than to help the other person.

Both partners are seen together as soon as possible in the family home. They are told what we can offer in terms of social support, for pain management and family counselling. At this time they are asked which medical practitioners are involved and if those practitioners can be contacted to discuss co-operation. The family are usually expected to initiate this meeting. I will talk the family through the roles of these various practitioners so that I understand clearly what each practitioner does. This process also clarifies these functions for the family. Most of the following interventions take place in the home of the patient.

Once practitioners are contacted and their permission gained to work with the family then I contact those practitioners to discuss what is to happen next. In the cases of hospital treatment, my access to specialist consultation is informal and often occurs during routine visits with the patient for treatment, e.g. while platelets are being replaced.

For the general practitioner either consent is given because the family doctor knows me already, or the general practitioner comes out to see how I practise. This is a reflection of the genuine desire of some practitioners to learn about 'complementary' practice.

Priests do not have this problem and have direct access to families. However, I believe that rather than work in parallel with the family doctor they could offer to work in harmony.

Who is family?

The family are asked who in the family would help in time of need and in terms of general support. The concept of 'family' varies from family to family. Some people have an '**instrumental**' concept of family. These family members are those who could be called upon for quite specific activities: i.e. distant relatives may be appropriate for telephone conversations to talk over difficulties and who would be seen as 'close'. At the same time there are geographically close relatives who can be used for transport but who are not seen as 'close family'.

It is important to emphasize, particularly with young couples, that they have to be clear what they are asking family members for, and not to expect that somehow their family will 'know' what they need. Part of my work is to help people identify their needs and then to be able to state them clearly. For example I saw a young woman recently who needed her family's help to do her weekly shopping. The round of hospital visits, sleepless nights, home 'nursing' and child-minding was beginning to take its toll. However, her parents seemed to be oblivious of her needs. She had to cope, and they believed she was coping. Once she worked out a way of asking them to take her into town, to wait for her while she shopped, and then to bring her home her life became less fraught. She achieved this without having 'not to cope'. This may seem quite trivial but it met **her need** as she expressed it. By being clear about these needs she could begin to clarify other needs and ask for them to be met.

Other families are far more '**sentimental**' in their construing of 'family'. In this way any one who is involved with these families on a regular basis, who visits regularly and who listens to problems is 'family'. I am adopted into such networks on the grounds of regular listening. Any such person becomes temporarily 'one of the family'. While these families are easy to work with in that I feel accepted into a loving community, there is a pitfall. When I become involved in this way then I have to accept that all the emotions involved with grief and bereavement will manifest themselves in me too. We cannot become part of a family and stay separate. This may sound dreadfully 'unprofessional' to some counsellors. However, what these families ask for is love and commitment in a way which they can understand. Once you decide not to withhold that commitment then be aware of the consequences. It is because of these consequences that I advocate supervision, or spiritual guidance, for counsellors, as you will see in the final chapter.

A third group of families are '**restricted**'. They are tightly knit with a small membership. Their boundaries are drawn around the marital pair and the children (regardless of age or geographical distance). Their perspective is to 'get by without too much outside help.' Any help is inevitably outside and we must be careful when working with these families that we listen carefully to their needs and do not overstep the boundaries that they set. Friends, however, are seen as separate from the family. These families are predominantly professional and express great store on being autonomous. When working with them it is an act of love to curb our helpful eagerness such that we temper our desires to their needs.

Family membership appears to be a function of 'instrumentality', i.e. those who can carry out particular supporting functions. This instrumentality is modified by 'sentimentality', i.e. by a willingness to make a benevolent and fraternal contact with the family. Close friends can attain the status of family membership by fulfilling particular functions. For the 'restricted' families most of their needs are met by their self-sufficiency.

Family	**Membership**	**Permeability**
restricted	few members	restricted outside help
instrumental	variable membership	selective outside help
sentimental	expansive membership	open to outside help

These distinctions are important in helping such families. By discovering the style of families it is possible to offer help which can be accepted.

For example, with 'instrumental families' it is possible to define the help offered in terms of specific functions such as counselling, pain relief, child-minding. For 'sentimental families' the initial approach is made and delivered in terms of social contact, of attending large family meetings and using the resources of family structure to provide emotional support and practical help.

In 'restricted' families it is important to tread carefully and avoid overtones of welfare. These families in some ways are handicapped by their self-sufficiency in that their contacts for support are few. However, they do understand professional roles and respond to such an approach. The skill lies in promoting permeability of the family boundary whereby social support can be accepted without the family perceiving themselves as becoming '**dependent**'.

Family change

The sources of distress in the families are located in the interaction of the physical, psychological, social and spiritual changes. In working with the patient in the context of the family it is possible to meet the needs not only of the person who is dying but also of the survivors. In some ways the process of handling death is a preparation for handling life for those who remain.

There are two properties in the course of dying. One is that death takes place over time. Death can be quick or slow, but there is always a process of dying. Second, the course of death has a shape. A person can steadily decline and then meet a sudden end, or after an initial acute episode may linger on for several months. Whether this course of dying is seen as a lingering death and tragic loss, or an opportunity to resolve existential issues and prepare for a future, depends very much upon the family's construing of death and the input of external support.

There are critical junctures during this process where it is possible to meet the needs of the family. Some practitioners see the main approach of working with families where there is cancer as being one of crisis management. If critical junctures are appreciated then there is less need of 'crisis' work. An understanding of process and available resources means that plans can be made which are not responsive to sudden events but to expected incidents. Similarly, by encouraging a regular community contact then crises are contextualized within the routine activity of friendship.

The first important point of contact is when a diagnosis is made. It is at such a time when families can be met and talked with and a format worked out for visiting the family at home and contacting other professionals. Much of my work at this time is spent in working out strategies for gaining more information for the patients from the medical practitioners. Note that this approach does not necessarily imply that I gather the information from those practitioners personally, or have a comprehensive knowledge of terminal illness. The emphasis is on supporting family members in their efforts to ask questions and find out more for themselves. The process of discovery itself gives the family some control over their activities.

One way of supporting the family is to go through their last hospital interview, discover what they understand, and then discuss the questions that understanding raises. These questions can then be written down and asked at the next consultation.

Some families want to read about their problem and it is useful to have a library of resource material to meet such needs.

Hospital appointments can be times of difficulty. Throughout a career of illness these important junctures deliver information about the efficacy of treatment and always include decisions about what to do next. As the illness progresses there is a lack of certainty when attempts at treatment fail. Not only is there a sense of diminishing control but also the realization and anticipation of physical deterioration and death. This is often exacerbated by the debilitating effects of the treatment itself.

At these times it is important to meet with families after appointments and discuss issues of:

(a) the awareness of death, disintegration and loss of self;
(b) the anticipation of pain and the implications for pain management;
(c) the physical sequelae of both treatment and the disease process and their management (nausea, incontinence, change in physical appearance, anorexia);
(d) the expression of frustration, helplessness, anxiety and depression;

(e) the change in family roles and structure during the process of dying and after death;
(f) the future welfare of the family after death (financial and social);
(g) the spiritual and existential questions raised at this time about the nature of suffering (feeling of being abandoned by God, guilt about past deeds or ideas of punishment).

All of these issues have ramifications for the rest of the family. Feelings of hopelessness are not necessarily limited to the patient. The management of pain and the basic nursing of the patient are often managed at home by a spouse. Pain is not only an internal response to tissue damage; it is an experience which exists within an emotional and relational context. If a spouse is elderly or ailing then a family member who has left home is often asked to help. This process of returning home and managing a different role within the family can be difficult.

Nursing and the physical support of the patient can mean a change in relationships within the family. A former breadwinner has to become dependent and this can challenge both the personal identity of the patient and that of other family members. This causes particular difficulty when medication is used for pain relief, or the patient becomes so debilitated that the process of decision-making changes.

> *For example*: In one family I saw, the husband decided that to gain his wife's attention he would ring a bell by his bedside. His wife was then expected to attend to him. When she did not he became distressed. His distress was not only related to his lack of ability to cope with his increasing physical problems but also with the understanding that his wife was taking over more and more activities and making more and more decisions within the home. This was not an attempt to wrest power from her husband but a reflection of the burgeoning demands upon her time. Time to sit and debate over decisions was seen as a luxury and a painful reflection of his loss of his abilities. This loss was painful for both partners and signified a change in the relationship. A long and fruitful life together became truncated and the immediate future appeared to be filled with difficulty and distress.

This particular problem was handled with humour. Once the patient was perceived as 'Quasimodo' and his wife as 'Esmeralda' (from Victor Hugo's *The Hunchback of Notre Dame)*, then 'the bells, the bells' took on a different connotation.

The expression of dissatisfaction was also used as an opportunity to discuss the loss of physical potency. Although this discussion took place with both partners together it stemmed from separate interviews with each partner. When sexual activity becomes painful or impossible it is possible to encourage partners to lie together and hold each other. The maintenance and encouragement of intimacy is important at a time of impending isolation and loneliness.

The experience of dying raises many spiritual questions (as shown above). What was previously unasked, or only vaguely formulated, gains an immediacy. At these times both the person and the family can find themselves without the spiritual tools, if you like, of thought and prayer to discover answers to their questions. Some people have not been aware of a need to maintain their spiritual development, and dying highlights that lack. It is at these times that priests and lay persons can teach both directly and indirectly. Praying with someone and allowing them to voice their own prayers is an important activity in this process. At these times it is important to avoid any condemnation of the person for their seeming neglect either in what you say, in what you do, or more importantly, within your own heart. When people are dying they come face to face with all the things that they have neglected to do in their lives. We must be willing to accept them as they are. It is not part of our ministry to judge.

Relief and comfort

Other than the negotiation of family changes the principal area of work is that of bringing comfort and relief. Many of the interventions used are specific to the person experiencing the pain, but are made in the presence of other family members. Simply interspersing the conversation with words of 'comfort' and 'relief' is an intervention in itself.

By distracting attention from pain, and using words of comfort we can help to alleviate pain. Please note that I am not advocating these approaches only. Medication is important. The constant emphasis is upon 'what works most effectively'. This includes the experience of side-effects. Meditation can have negative side-effects if a person continues to struggle with a technique at the expense of ignoring effective medication!

Pain relief is not confined to the body of the patient, it extends throughout the body of the family.

> *For example*: The author was asked to see a woman who had a continuing pain in the right side of her body. This woman was taught a number of relaxation techniques, introduced to meditation and encouraged to use self-hypnosis.
>
> Each of these sessions was recorded on audiotape for the person to use at any time for the relief of pain, and for gathering strength to face the day. However, various family members would attend these sessions. The reason they gave for this was that they gained their own comfort and relief from using the techniques, and from knowing that the patient was gaining relief too.

The main reasons for using such methods for pain relief are:

(a) to avoid the confusion and drowsiness, and other side-effects, of some medication;
(b) to avoid the memory of pain by using amnesia;

(c) to limit the anxiety of a future threatening event; and
(d) to bring sleep or rest.

These techniques are not used as replacements for medication but as complementary approaches. With medication there is always a trade-off between pain relief and consciousness. By using both together it is possible to keep patients alert and responsive while removing the experience of pain. The effect upon the family is that they no longer see a loved one suffering and, perhaps as importantly, that loved one is not as irritable when rested and pain-free.

Of course not all practitioners will have access to these techniques. However, it is possible to introduce therapists with these techniques to such families, and encourage other practitioners in the network to work in this way.

In my practice meditation, visualization, hypnosis and relaxation are all used for strengthening the patient's resolve, bringing hope, relieving boredom and rehearsing difficult future events. This is done in the context of the family. Family members are encouraged to be present. At each session each person present is asked what needs to be focused on during that session. By using an audiotape and encouraging self-reliance the therapeutic contact is minimized and the patient given some control over their problems. Such techniques allow the patient and the family to have a choice of alternatives.

Some of these concepts like 'hope' may seem rather vague. However, it is these issues which are raised by families. If we are to be involved in healing we must be responsive to such problems. It is important that we do not dodge these existential issues either out of ignorance or a desire for simplicity of practice which is concerned solely with symptomatic relief. It is tackling some of these problems which brings relief.

For example: A woman was in the late stages of cancer. Her general practitioner had terminated her hospital treatment because the treatment was hastening her death faster than the course of the disease. The woman and her husband were both worn out by the management of her pain and the constant round of hospital visits. The main problem presented by this family was that the woman, when she woke up in the morning, could not face the day itself after a largely sleepless night. She had lost the will to live. By using meditation, prayer and visualization techniques this woman discovered a resource within herself which gave her some comfort.

As a secondary problem her husband, the general practitioner and the parish priest were concerned that she was not talking about her impending death with them. They would talk to her about many things in her daily life but then go outside the house to discuss her slow decline and whether or not to tell her that she was dying.

By talking to the practitioner, the husband, the priest and the patient

> together the issue of dying was addressed. The woman was simply told of the concern of the men in her life that she was dying and not being given the opportunity to talk about it. Her reply was that she knew that she was dying but was more concerned with 'living' to the full the days she had remaining with her family and children. This gave me an opportunity to talk to the priest and the husband about their difficulties in facing her death.

In everything this woman tried her family would come and listen. While concentrating on her as a patient other members could be free to join in. After the first session, when I introduced a relaxation technique to promote rest, both her husband and mother asked to sit in on the sessions, not to scrutinize me, but for the benefit they gained for themselves, and to learn the technique.

The result was a creative use by these family members of relaxation techniques. Her mother used it to gain rest while sitting with her daughter at night. Her husband used it for calming himself down before hospital visits with the consultant oncologist, and after his wife's death when he thought he could not cope with the children.

The main emphasis in this way of working is to develop a family culture where needs can be expressed and where the family can learn to formulate their own solutions to problems. This includes a culture of prayer where spiritual needs can be voiced, and a belief that they will be heard and answered. From this culture it is also possible to develop resources which are already present rather than seek for, or assume, pathology in family relationships. Families are seen as having strengths which can be promoted, rather than being inept or incapable. It is a trap for us to pretend that we can know what they know, or that we have skills which they do not have access to.

> *For example*: In a family recently they prayed for pain relief in the later stages of a painful illness. Later that same day, the general practitioner 'dropped in' on an informal visit. On seeing their distress he prescribed the appropriate medication which he had been reluctant to prescribe before. This family believed that a prayer was answered.

Family process and cancer

Many families are concerned that in some way they may be guilty for the patient developing a terminal illness. The modern understandings which stress lifestyle influences, personality factors and marital and family relationships can place a burden on the family. The family then begin to search for a cause. The hope remains that the identification of a cause may bring the possibility of a solution. To be confronted with the idea that cancer is caused by difficulties and conflict in a marriage, or a lack of faith, is debilitating.

Blame hinders healing. If we follow a Christ who is all compassion then blame has no place in our repertoire of explanations. Similarly, advice which is misinformed medically, psychologically and spiritually is damaging. When we do not know it is best to say that we do not know. Not only is it true, but also removes us from the omnipotent stance of having to know everything. This too can be a form of teaching.

Some authors, while suggesting that family relationships may influence the onset of disease and the course of the illness, emphasize that as yet there is no causal connection between family functioning and the onset of cancer. Certainly the family functions as a system in relation to the physical illness and adapts to dying in its own particular way. Rigidity of structure may inhibit the influence of others who wish to offer support, but it is a fanciful step to say that such rigidity is influential in causing illness. Similarly psychological studies have found no reliable evidence to support a correlation between psychological processes and cancer. It has been suggested that suppressed anger in women under fifty years of age may be implicated in breast cancer, and this has ramifications for their primary relationships. Of these women we would ask 'Angry with whom: themselves, their families, their spouses, their doctor or God?' However, as yet, *no* satisfactory scientific evidence exists. The only real evidence about the causes of cancer are those linked to cigarette smoking, food additives and environmental factors. The shift of emphasis away from these factors onto personal relationships is a political move.

There may be a certain sort of interaction which is a sufficient condition for the onset of disease concurrent with other causal factors, i.e. genetics and environmental factors (viruses and carcinogens). Or it may be that some patterns of family interaction are sensitizing or predisposing influences. One form of interaction may interfere with the body's functions of healing and resistance while another may facilitate these. As yet we have no adequate knowledge.

We can begin to look at how the disease is currently a problem. This is the position taken in this chapter. No past causes are assumed. The primary area of focus is the present, and how family difficulties are handled. To work in this way sidetracks any issue of blame. The family are encouraged to participate if invited by the patient and the patient's spouse. Problem handling between all participants, lay, familial, communal and professional is co-operative and not competitive.

Social activity and support

By using a community network the family can be supported without the intrusion of too many professionals. A common feature seems to be that on the diagnosis of a life-threatening illness, or the development of worsening and publicly evident symptoms, the family reduce their social contacts. Sometimes friends simply stop visiting.

In this practice the family are encouraged to join the home groups mentioned in an earlier chapter. These are held regularly in a person's home and are not set up specifically for the support of the patient but are for the encouragement of nurturing relationships within the community. Each group is different. Some groups have a set format and discuss issues. Other groups are social. The patient and their family are encouraged to make friends or develop old acquaintances. From these contacts friendships grow and the family are open to being visited at home. All of this is under the control of the patient and the family. No person is coerced to join a group.

A man who became a close friend of mine said that the knowledge that one could make a friendship, although in the process of dying, helped him to make sense of dying. In this way the formal sacrament of the body and blood of Christ was reflected in the loving friendship of our families sharing a meal together. Our Christianity becomes a living faith. Our spiritual food is shared.

Another way that families are supported, and which uses this home group contact, is the celebration of the sacrament of the Eucharist in the family home. The format used for these services is described in the chapter on home visiting. It is important to remember that the initial referral for help is through church contacts. The parish priest attends to the spiritual needs of the patient and family, prays with them regularly and guides them in their reading if requested. Once a month friends and family, according to the wishes of the patient and their family, gather together in the patient's home to celebrate the sacrament of the Eucharist together. This is one more tie into a network of support. It is an activity which allows people to share their common faith but also to express their common concerns.

The friendships forged during these activities are helpful in the short-term support of the patient and the family, but are significantly important in the long-term support of the survivors.

Bereavement

When death occurs much of the therapeutic support ends. Grief and bereavement are not situations for therapeutic management either. However, the ties and links of friendship are appropriate at the time of the funeral and in supporting the family in their grief. These links of friendship endure. In my experience the continuing support of the survivors is managed not therapeutically but informally by the naturalistic means of friendship in a context of community. It is here where the vital relationships continue, where the visits are maintained, and when the prayers can still be offered.

This context of community is structured initially. Groups have to be set up and then co-ordinated. People can be guided to appropriate groups. All the groups are introduced to the notion of problems being contextualized by family process. However, it must be emphasized that these groups are not set up specifically for the dying and their families. They are set up for mutual support and teaching where people can get together socially. They are used as a vehicle for the support of families at a later date, and are used generally to support those people who do feel isolated or lonely.

Community support in this form is based on the idea of mutuality. No person is referred to a group for support as such but invited to join a group for their own benefit and the support of others. These groups are not run by professionals, although occasionally someone may be invited to address a group or share a cup of coffee. As these groups endure there are inevitably widows and widowers who can support and show understanding to new members whose spouses are dying. In this way expertise is not resident in one person but becomes a communal attribute.

Co-ordination of support

For any parish or community worker working in this way a truly systemic perspective needs to be adopted. It is necessary to understand the interlocking systems of the individual, the marital, the familial and the communal.

Most of my preliminary work and a large part of the continuing work is in co-ordinating other professionals and community initiatives. The most important understanding we can have here is that of boundary. Professionals often have clearly defined tasks and are happy to work with others who have complementary roles with clearly defined tasks. This definition is not always apparent with lay helpers, and as co-ordinator it is important to negotiate a clarity of understanding about what helpers can do. Boundaries do not have to restrict. They can be used to allow us freedom of movement, and in that balance between freedom and constraint we can allow others to do their healing work.

Of course it is inappropriate to define or limit friendship. It is appropriate, however, to suggest that too many 'counsellors' with differing aims can make things worse, or at least introduce confusion at a time of uncertainty. It is possible for friends in the grip of their own grief or frustration to interfere in a way which is counter-productive. To avoid this I have concentrated on identifying tasks with professionals and then meeting with families and friends to determine who is doing what. A by-product of this is that one person can see where activities are being duplicated. I must emphasize that friendships must continue, and that we must remain committed with the whole of our being. By recognizing what each person can do then we allow our love to serve others rather than ourselves.

Following on from this, there are times when it is appropriate to restrict access to the family. Sometimes the needs of nursing have to take precedence and it is the presence of a person with a long-term and comprehensive picture of what is happening who can make such a decision.

For example: A friend was dying and his physical needs were becoming more and more demanding. Both his wife and the nursing sister from the hospital were attending him through the night. On hearing of his imminent death many people wished to see him and say goodbye. Each person was concerned to minister to him in his time of need. However, being visited is a very taxing business, particularly if you are meeting the needs of others too. It was necessary to ask some people not to visit as the patient was becoming weaker and weaker. In this case it was the specialist nurse, who was not only a friend but had a wide range of experience and skills, who made the decision about visiting. It was a measure of our strength as a loving community to abdicate our personal preferences to her knowledge. Similarly, it was important to stress the need for the family to spend time together and for the professionals to withdraw.

In contacting other professionals it is important to be clear about what we say we can do and make sure that we say it in terms that they understand. Medical practitioners realize the need for counselling. There is some hesitancy on their part about the use of hypnosis, visualization techniques, prayer or anointing. This hesitancy disappears if we take time either to demonstrate or to discuss exactly what we do. All these activities are part of building a system for further interventions with other families. Similarly, they may not be sure of what we do when we talk of celebrating the Eucharist or the laying on of hands.

The initial months of this practice were spent with practitioners as much as with families. Once practitioners understood what I was doing, and I understood them, then working together became easier.

By the same token I have presented this way of working to a number of practitioner and community groups. This enables the idea of co-operative work to become part of the culture. By working with our communities and promoting understanding then we can begin to work together. It is the indirect contact which can open the door to personal contacts. This has led to a wider source of referrals for problems other than terminal illness, and from people who have no church ties. What people say attracts them to this way of working is that it is compassionate and has no overtones of welfare. They also appreciate being consulted about their problem; and they can say what they want to without fear of condemnation because of their ignorance or because of what they feel. I hear a lot of expressed hostility some of which results from unfeeling and misdirected advice, and some of which is a reflection of impotence in the face of a crisis. By offering acceptance then we teach others to accept. By forgiving we promote forgiveness.

Conclusion

It is necessary to have an understanding of family structure, family life-cycle changes and boundary in co-ordinating a community response to helping families with cancer.

The characteristics of this service are:

(1) An holistic perspective which is concerned with developing comprehensive programmes to meet the physical, psychological, social and spiritual needs of those who come for help.
(2) Programmes which are responsive to family style and promote family coping mechanisms and strengths. Self-care and education are emphasized before treatment and dependence.
(3) A way of working which stresses practitioner co-operation and utilizes lay networks.
(4) Pharmacological and surgical remedies are contextualized within personal, relational and familial interventions.
(5) An active partnership is encouraged between care-givers and consumers.
(6) Change as a process is accepted and understood as having ramifications for all family members. Crises are anticipated at critical junctures in the process of dying.
(7) Continuity of care is seen as extending beyond the death of the patient and is contained within the realm of informal community support.
(8) Communication with other professionals and community groups is seen as important in fostering the development of such a service.
(9) An emphasis is placed on linking the celebration of the formal sacraments of the Eucharist and healing with living a Christian life of love, compassion, prayer, kindness, friendship, gentleness, with the many becoming one body.

7 *Reaching Out: Healing in Practice*

The practice of healing involves a sensitivity to the multiple needs of others. Of course we feel daunted when we attempt to reconcile all the varying realms of human experience which include the physical, the psychological, the social and the spiritual. Yet we do it all the time. We balance many aspects of our lives without having to be constantly aware of what we are doing. Occasionally we overwork ourselves, or confuse 'busyness' with effectiveness, and use solutions which are inappropriate. We become unaware.

In the way of working described here we have to be aware of ourselves and others. We also have to trust that if we pray and reflect then our actions will incorporate the wholeness we seek and our own awareness will be developed. Listening to ourselves is an important part of listening to others. All too often we neglect God speaking to us through our own inner voice. If we neglect this voice how can we hear God speaking through the voices of others? In this way stillness and listening with an awareness of ourselves is not negative self-regard but an awareness of our own potential. This potential incorporates our own weakness as well as our strength. By promoting our self-awareness we realize how we encourage, or interrupt, the process of the Spirit working within us.

In the following examples I hope to demonstrate how some of the endeavours in the previous chapters have been incorporated into the healing ministry. These will include individual, family and community approaches. None are separate, all are interconnected. The names have been changed to maintain anonymity.

Sue

Sue was a young woman with two young children. Her husband had been given time off work to look after her. The problem she faced was that the chemotherapy and radiotherapy she was receiving for the treatment of her cancer were proving to be dangerous. As her condition worsened, her general practitioner asked that all treatment be stopped and suggested that she had no further contact with the consultant oncologist. Sue felt like giving in and the whole family were distressed, demoralized and exhausted. All those involved were angry about the lack of support that Sue had received, and the way in which the treatment had been isolated from the whole perspective of family life.

In the terms of the previous chapter this was a 'sentimental' family who welcomed others into their circle. At the first visit the sacraments of healing were administered and the Eucharist celebrated. Her mother and husband were present and shared in the service. I talked to her about the use of visualization and meditation, and gave her an introductory tape which demonstrated a relaxation technique and focused on inner healing (see Chapter 3). This allowed her to try out procedures in the privacy of her own home, in her own time and under her own control.

Taped recordings of interventions are an important part of my work. They are always tailored to the specific needs of the person, and the family if necessary. I use a general tape introduction but also like to have made some contact with the person involved before they are given the tape. If I cannot meet the person with the problem I like the person who is giving the tape to have a close relationship with the listener. To give out tapes as a universal panacea is to miss the whole point of healing which lies in the relationship of one person with another. It is all too easy to give out a tape, and miss out the stages of listening and loving. It would be possible to produce a whole number of tapes for specific clinical problems. All we would have to do is match the tape with the problem. To do so would be to fall into the trap into which medicine sometimes falls: treating the disease rather than the person.

Therapeutic tasks

At the second visit, which Sue arranged through her husband's instigation, I concentrated on particular tasks.

(1) Anxiety

Sue was concerned about her own anxiety for the future, her inability to rest, and lack of hope. I developed a countdown technique with her (see Chapter 3) which concentrated on her being filled with light. This also helped to regulate her breathing by encouraging her to breathe deeply into her body. She was encouraged to find a quiet place within herself which became a haven of personal strength for her and was used as a resource from which to contemplate the future.

(2) Visualization

At this visit she asked particularly to be able to move her hand. Her arm had become paralysed as a result of the previous treatment. The reasons she gave for wanting to gain the use of her hand were that she could hold her children, and would have some sign of her body being able to recover.

The technique used was to visualize light streaming from a candle along the neural pathways within her body until in her own mind's eye she could see light streaming from her fingers. Her fingers began to move. For Sue this was a sign of real hope. It was also a thrill for her husband to witness this movement as he sat with both of us.

This session was taped using a portable tape recorder and a lapel microphone. Sue could play back this tape whenever she needed it. Throughout the following months we made a series of tapes appropriate to particular problems. What emerges from this way of working is that the willingness to sit down with someone and try to help is in itself a comfort. To have some resource, such as a tape, which promotes well-being in the midst of turmoil and degeneration is a message of hope and love in the world.

(3) Recalling a time of strength

I also used a technique learned from neuro-linguistic programming. Neuro-linguistic programming assumes that what we say to a person can influence their bodily processes. There is a cautionary note in this. If we believe that what we say influences people then we had better be careful what we say to everyone we meet in everyday life. In a way we know this already. If we are hostile then others suffer pain.

Sue was encouraged to recall a time when she felt at her strongest and most creative and to allow these feelings to flood through her body. Similarly she was asked to recall how she moved and thought at such a time and asked to allow these thoughts and movements to locate themselves within herself and influence her current state. By introducing a light touch of the hand on her wrist when she felt at her strongest it was possible for her to allow her husband to touch her wrist and invoke this strength whenever she needed it. By encouraging a technique of touch which her husband could use then he was involved directly in helping her. It is important for therapists not to become surrogate husbands/wives or to usurp the role of comforter. Spouses often feel helpless at such times. Helpers by their very willingness to help must be wary of pushing the spouse into a peripheral role. The deepening of the relationship betweeen husband and wife at such times is of paramount importance not only for the healing of the patient, but for the relationship and the *future* of the spouse who remains.

(4) Comfort and relief

During the recording of the tape I interspersed the flow of words with suggestions of comfort and relief. The recovery of sensation was proposed as a tide which would return in the cyclical nature of the world. At times this tide would ebb and many hidden things would be revealed. At other times there would be a flow of comfort and she would gain relief. I used her language, literally the words she used, about regaining her strength and use of her hand and the flow of strength within her body to that hand. Learning the language of another person is an act of love. To use their words is a demonstration, albeit indirectly, that we have truly listened to them.

(5) Imagery

For the cancer in her back I used a technique of imagery where the growth was visualized as ice. She was sitting on a beach allowing the heat from the sun to dissolve the ice. It is important to note here that I had checked carefully whether she used visual images, sounds or feelings in her imagination. Some people are visualizers in terms of pictures. However, some people are verbalizers and imagine in words or sounds. They literally hear things in their heads and carry on internal dialogues. Some people are kinesthetic. They imagine in terms of sensation and feelings. Sue used visual images and feelings. She also enjoyed sitting in the sun so this visualization was attached to a realm of experience which she had already experienced. This is an important point. If we listen to the language people use, the style of that language, and to the experiences they have had, then we can begin to communicate with them at a very deep level.

At a later visit I constructed a tape which used an image technique where Sue climbed a mountain on an uphill struggle. When exhausted she was to look up and find she was at the summit and from there could begin to discern the purpose of the struggle. This was done in the presence of other family members who by now had come along to the session to find out what I was doing. They said that they all gained much relief from this exercise. I used the metaphor of the Spirit which leads us on as a guide when we are lost, and who strengthens us when we are weary.

Her general practitioner sat in on a session and approved of what I was doing. Another technique I used with Sue when she felt that nothing made sense, apart from prayer, was to imagine that she held the sky in one hand. She was to focus on that sky, breathing deeply until the clouds cleared. This was an attempt to introduce a technique whereby she would not hurry herself on too quickly and to allow her body to catch up with her thoughts.

(6) Prayer

I also laid on hands and prayed with her and her husband together for what they identified as appropriate issues. It is important to concentrate on the content of these prayers and reflect accurately what people ask for. However, beyond the content is a deeper and more fundamental issue. Two married people were praying together and becoming further united in their love. I was privileged to be part of that, and therein lies my own healing too. We are not separate. Messages would also be sent around the prayer chain for prayer at times of difficulty, or for prayers of thanksgiving.

Ministering to friends

During the months that followed there were many sessions and tape recordings. The children would come in from school during a session and nonchalantly say 'hello', or later sit and listen. Family members or friends would be present. Sue ministered to their needs. They told her of their problems. She listened, told them of her understandings, and loved them. In the way in which she faced death others saw their own mortality. What she offered to them was a real experience of God's love for all of us. She was not abandoned. In all that she did she demonstrated a woman coping with pain and loss with dignity and at peace.

Eventually she had a massive chest infection and died. She died peacefully in the arms of her husband. To have met Sue during these last months was to know about healing. There was no miraculous cure, but many miraculous moments. There was a turn around from despair to hope, from dying to living, and from anguish to peace. Her family came to terms with her dying, and her children were helped to understand. Here was the healing. How easy it would have been to miss if we had insisted on a cure as the only evidence of healing!

I always try to attend the funeral. It is important for my own process of grieving as much as it is for the family and friends. All too often we can escape into our therapeutic roles and hide behind a professional barrier, or the role of carer. To do so is to engage in a process of gradual desensitization. If we separate ourselves from those with whom we work, the very qualities of openness and sensitivity in the face of loss which we need to develop are denied and wither.

George

I first saw George in hospital at the instigation of the parish priest and after first checking with George's wife that she had no objections. I talked with her indirectly about the difficulties facing the families of the chronic sick. George had chronic myeloid leukaemia.

George suggested that the visit be in hospital. We discussed hypnosis as a means of pain management and for strengthening his resolve. He regarded hypnotherapy as a useful therapeutic tool. I gave him a pre-recorded tape to use in the hospital simply to prepare him for the sound of my voice and as a precursor to any therapeutic interventions. Ironically he used it within those first few days to gain some sleep, and to rest from the busy atmosphere of the ward. I had not intended the tape to be used in such a way, but many people have told me since that the tape has that somnific effect. I suppose it is one way of saying my voice is boring without offending me!

Interventions

(1) Finding a source of strength

All the sessions were recorded on tape. A programme was set for six weeks, with set targets which included the maintenance of health and the development of physical, psychological and spiritual resources. I used the technique of neuro-linguistic programming described earlier to recall previous situations of strength.

(2) Imagery

George was continually encouraged to realize the flow of healing within himself by using several exercises. One was to go deep within himself to a control room. Once there he would identify the wiring circuitry and see which circuits were connected, and those which were malfunctional. Then he was to reconnect those circuits until all systems were functional. He imagined that all the lights on his internal control panel would glow green. As he had an abiding interest in electronics this imagery fitted into his own experience. As a general point in constructing such image techniques, it is important to listen to the patient and construct a solution which fits their frame of reference. George was also a gardener and this gave other possibilities for constructing image exercises for the promotion of growth and patience.

A difficulty which he faced, and which faces all cancer sufferers, is the struggle to carry on after the exhaustions of hospital treatment. Sometimes the round of hospital visits, tests, worry and daily living itself brings people to breaking-point. There seems no point to living, and it becomes an effort to start each day. This has an effect on their partners and their family. Do you push as a spouse, or do you let things go? Sometimes to push means to nag a loved one already in pain and distress. Then the carer becomes demoralized and loses his/her strength.

The technique I use here is the one I used with Sue. After an introductory relaxation I get the person to imagine climbing a hill, which gradually becomes a mountain. They have no reason for doing this other than that it is a journey which they find themselves on. The going gets tougher and the way steeper. What was at first a comfortable stroll becomes a slog. Their body is tired and they become dispirited. At the moment where they are about to give up they find themselves at the summit. Here they experience profound relief. From being at one moment exhausted, at the next they feel relief and begin to see a new vista. By encouragement to see, and feel, at such times they are led to their own understandings. I believe that this is far more ecologically sound than attempting to give them words of comfort. They perceive. They know.

Prayer

There were regular sessions of prayer, the laying on of hands, and a celebration of the Eucharist within the home. At these intimate services family members were invited, or friends would visit. Somehow when people gather together in this way they open up the possibility of talking about difficult issues and for commenting on their own distress. By doing so they have access to alternative ways of handling that distress by the example of others. But, perhaps more importantly, there is the opportunity to speak out about that which is unspoken.

Getting on with life

After this initial six-week programme we met infrequently at his instigation. Generally I leave the instigation of contact in the hands of the person who needs help, or a family member. They ask when necessary. If a family member asks me to visit I visit them first, not the patient, unless the patient is too incapacitated to call.

There were signs of improvement, and George felt better. He went back to work briefly. During this time he had become impatient and irritable. He also 'knew' something was not quite right and could not put his finger on the problem. By using a visualization technique whereby he listened carefully to his own body systems he came to an awareness that his blood was not returning to normal. His inner fear was expressed outwardly. Although his white cell count had returned to normal following a bone-marrow graft, he failed to produce either red cells or platelets. His concern was that the residue of the cytotoxic drugs had killed off his precursor cells. This concern was proved to be correct. Not only did this give him confidence in his own awareness, but also demonstrated to me that we can know about our own bodies using these techniques. However, I do stress that it is important to have a companion or guide.

George needed a second bone-marrow graft and we worked on the process of supporting him and his family psychologically and spiritually through that series of harrowing procedures. This meant working in harmony with the hospital team who were not only patient but compassionate in their treatment of the family. It would be a mistake to think that we, as Christians, have a monopoly on compassion. It was in the working together, and these introductory dialogues, where the later strength to persevere and the platform for healing were developed.

Projection

One of the problems George's wife Janet faced was that people kept expecting her to 'break down' and cry. They would talk to her and tell her that she could cry if she wanted to, they would not mind. At this time those friends were also expressing their concern to me that Janet was not crying. As Janet said, 'There were too many things to be done, life has to carry on'. What appeared to be happening was that friends were projecting their own feelings of distress on to Janet. It wasn't that Janet did not feel. In her conversations with me she expressed her fears and difficulties. It was simply that she did not give others the opportunity to express their emotions through her. This would have been an additional burden, and too much to bear. There are no templates for coping. What we can offer others is to support their style of coping and not impose upon them our own coping strategies.

Similarly Janet was reluctant to talk about any long-term plans. Her plans were for the short term. Some thought that this was shortsighted on her part. Once again it is important to remember that we cannot give others our sense of prescience, or our wishful thinking. The challenge for George's and Janet's friends was that the prognosis for this type of chronic leukaemia was poor, and they would have to struggle with that understanding just as George and Janet had. There is a danger that reading books on healing is taken as a substitute for real-life experience. It was easier to retreat into the comfortable stories of healing works rather than to face the realities of daily Christian living which included both hope and despair. However, for a while the second graft took. George returned to teaching and part-time practice.

Dying

This optimism faded. George was dying, and he was only given a short time to live: a matter of months or weeks. Janet called and asked me what she could tell people, and particularly the children. This was a period of preparatory and anticipatory grief. George was literally living on the blood of other people. We continued to visit to pray, to lay on hands, and to celebrate the Eucharist. The blood of Christ gained an extra significance in this context.

During this time we concentrated on meditations for the management of pain combined with the experience of acceptance. The medication for pain relief can cause unwanted side-effects, and the use of psychological techniques allows for less medication to be used initially. Some pain is organic and susceptible to medication, some is caused by anxiety and susceptible to other procedures. By using a combined approach it is possible to minimize the pharmacological interventions and some of the side-effects. Furthermore, the choice is placed in the hands of the patients who have a broader spectrum of responses to the management of their pain.

George and Janet spent a lot of time talking together and planning the future, for her support, and the support of their children. The way in which the children were told was planned beforehand according to the parents' perception of the children. This utilizes their own knowledge.

Simply by asking how they have delivered difficult information before is a useful starting place. The next thing is to ask what the best time and situation is, whether, for example, in their pyjamas before bed, cuddling up on the settee in the evening, or at a family meal with a treat to follow.

With more than one child it may be necessary to tell each child separately according to the parents' understanding of the child. Similarly, one parent may communicate such matters better to one child than the other. By careful listening it is possible to find an appropriate way of telling children which utilizes the residual strengths and abilities of the parents. This itself is a message to the parents that they have many hidden resources which they will be able to call upon in the future.

Change

Some authors see the process of dying as being divided into stages. Such a schema can be helpful as long as we remember that such schemata are metaphors for what takes place, and are not direct maps of reality. There are times when shock is clearly followed by denial, anger, depression, bargaining, acceptance and decathexis. When working with families it is possible to see these stages in different members at different times. Sometimes people will take it in turn to be angry. Rarely do people follow a textbook path.

The main issues for this couple centred around the changing role of parenting. There was a shift in the disciplining of the children and Janet had to assume the role of head of the household and begin to establish a pattern for the future. A further change of role was that from wife to nurse. The patience required to nurse another human being is taxing. When it is one's own spouse then it can promote many difficulties – particularly when a spouse is less reluctant to comply with difficult procedures, or is more complaining, than with a professional nurse.

To support George and his wife in the home the specialist nursing sister came from the hospital both to change his platelets and to nurse him at home. Once this happened, and it was known that she would be present right until the end, then she assumed an important primary role in George's management. This gave George and Janet another close confidant.

The tapes continued to be made concentrating on specific needs. Janet spent time simply holding George and comforting him. We continued to visit and celebrate in the home in the presence of invited guests. The prayer chain carried messages of support. Janet had joined a home group and was supported there, although she found it emotionally difficult. Friends would visit her and take her out shopping, and her parents came to stay regularly.

Eventually George died. His death was shared by the family. The children were aware of their father dying and this did cause consternation temporarily. However, they coped. They had a chance to talk with their father until the end. He told them what he most wanted to say to them, and they to him.

Barbara

Barbara had retired from her work. Her husband was still working although coming up to retirement age. Her children were all grown up and away from home. Three years previously she had had an operation for the removal of a cancer.

Her problem was that she was going blind in one eye. She had been told by her consultant that there was a 'growth' on her eye which was causing this progressive blindness. The prognosis was bleak. If the growth was benign she would go blind. If the growth was malignant then she would have to have the growth and the eye removed with the possibility of the cancerous cells spreading to secondary sites within her body.

As the reader can imagine she was anxious about the future and about any further medical contacts as she awaited an appointment with a specialist in London.

Interventions

(1) Prayer in the home

The first thing we did was to visit her at home and set up a pattern of home visiting. The format was always the same: a reading followed by the healing sacraments including anointing with oil. It was this foundation from which other interventions could be made. Again it was an attempt to meet her style of being in the world. Just as interventions with others had been informal this approach was formal. In this way we leave our needs for formality or informality and reach out to others.

(2) Targets

During these visits I carefully elicited her priorities of need and her style of talking about them, with specific targets for recovery. When we identify such targets then we know that someone has been healed.

(3) Tapes

After giving her an introductory tape I made a series of meditation tapes with her (see earlier in this chapter). She told me what she liked best, what she found helpful and what she wanted to focus on. Note the use of 'focus' for a woman who had problems with her sight. Ironically she was extremely adept at visualizing. My technique with her used light to dissolve her tumour such that it too was converted to particles of light which streamed from her.

These tapes were also used to bring relaxation and allay anxiety. One of her major fears was the forthcoming appointment and her ability to gather the necessary information at that appointment. Although as practitioners we know what we are saying, and may well give out information clearly, we forget that this information is often received in the context of distress. As I have said earlier much of my work concentrates on setting an agenda with the patient for the gathering of information and the seeking of clarity. Clarity at a time of confusion is itself a healing, and an aid to reducing anxiety.

The visit to London

The visits continued over the weeks, and we prayed in her home and in our prayer groups. When she saw the specialist he was surprised because the tests showed that the growth had halted. He had no reason to suggest why, other than that such growths can spontaneously stop growing. Barbara had a different explanation. She and her husband were overjoyed, and their account of the walk which they made in a London park afterwards will always remain with me as a powerful witness of thanksgiving. This was a couple in their sixties, not given to extravagant claims or overt expressions of charismatic gifts, yet they witnessed to the healing which they believed had happened in their lives. Their futures were transformed. Not only was her eye healed and her sight maintained, but their future together was healed. They were liberated once more from anxiety and possible pain to their loving marriage and an enjoyment of their retirement.

Harriet

We are often faced with marital problems in our roles as counsellors. My perspective on any problem is to locate it within the context of an intimate relationship. This does not mean that I blame either partner, or that all problems stem from difficult relationships. However, people live in intimate relationships and it is important to realize that, if we counsel one person and that counselling promotes change or maintains stability, there will be implications for those relationships. Occasionally we come across circumstances where the problem, although presented by an individual, is located within the context of a relationship. In the following study I will attempt to tease out some of the threads which run through this tapestry of relational conflict and the implications for healing.

Harriet was married with two children. She asked to see me for a marital problem which had been present over the past twelve years. This was a crisis appointment when the marital tension was at its greatest. Each family member was distressed. Her adolescent daughters were threatening to leave home or run away from school and her husband appeared to be 'depressed'. Harriet was in physical pain, worried, emotionally upset and concerned for her own sanity.

Although Harriet had received counselling previously, this had aimed at keeping her marriage together. The implication from those other counsellors, whom Harriet had seen, was that she was a weak-willed woman who was good-hearted but over-sensitive and making a lot of what was a small problem. In other words she was being told, as women often are when they complain, 'to put up and shut up'.

The marital conflict represented itself as her unwillingness to have sexual intercourse, as a lack of marital satisfaction, and a demand by her that she have an active role as a woman in her own right rather than occupy the role of 'housekeeper'. My understanding of the situation was that the advice she had received from other counsellors had been normative, overly prescriptive and sexist. Normative in that she was implicitly being asked to settle back into the role of wife and mother which denied her own personality, and her needs. Prescriptive because she was constantly given 'good' advice about what to do when she was perfectly capable of reaching her own decisions. This advice may not have been as overt as 'do this then do that', but part of a guidance which led her to particular conclusions which were based on a platform of marital reconciliation. I am not against reconciliation, but that reconciliation has to be on mutually acceptable grounds, otherwise we have people – usually women – living out their lives in distress and pain. This advice was sexist in the implication that she was making a lot of her problem, being 'rebellious' and emotional. In short she refused to co-operate with therapeutic interventions which were based on attempts to change her rather than the relationship.

Interventions

(1) Acceptance

I listened to her assuming that she was a responsible mature woman who had a whole range of natural human desires and needs which were not being fulfilled. My perspective was that she was a strong, capable women performing the difficult task of being a wife, mother and person in her own right. Furthermore I believed that she was legitimate in the demands that she was making and that she was acting in good faith. This was acceptance of her as a person and is a cornerstone of the work of healing.

(2) Stay constant and allow others to change

She was given a task to carry out over the six weeks following the interview, but only after she had asked what to do. This task was to maintain one constant position for six weeks, neither leaving nor moving closer. The position adopted was that she would offer to see a marital or family counsellor and would invite her husband to attend. This was a reflection of her own solution. Although I was being prescriptive I was prescribing Harriet's own solution gleaned during the conversation. Once again this is a process of affirmation, albeit indirect.

The issue of separation or divorce was to be handled by her as and when she thought necessary. When, or if, she told the children was to be based on her knowledge of them. Once again this validated her own knowledge as a mother about her own children, rather than implying that her needs for fulfilment would damage her daughters.

My view on marital counselling is that, when a couple – or an individual – comes to me for help, then I am willing either to talk about their coming together or to help them separate. As a Christian this poses a dilemma as I am helping to split a marriage which is apparently united by God. However, as a therapist I know that the more we try and keep some people together the more they struggle to part. If we help some people to achieve an emotional distance so that they can appreciate each other then they sometimes come together. The difficulty arises if we have a hidden agenda for unity which contradicts their hidden agenda to separate. Sometimes people do not know if they want to go or stay, but they know that living together is painful. A period of neutrality without having to make binding decisions about the future is an important step in the process of reconciliation. Reconciliation may mean estrangement as husband and wife, but an amicable arrangement for the continuing relationship of parenting.

(3) Small goals

Harriet set her own goals for change. Her demands on her husband and children were small and reasonable. But importantly those demands were presented in such a way that she could maintain them without wavering. Her position in the relationship was to be one of stability and consistency. By making small demands they could see her as firm and resolute no matter what they did to upset her equilibrium. They might shout, cry, curse or cajole but she would continue to state her position firmly and clearly. This was only for six weeks. By remaining resolute she could enable them to change.

(4) See a doctor

She was also encouraged to check her physical symptoms with her doctor. Although they may have been emotional, as she suggested, it was most important to have the symptoms investigated. This she did, and was satisfied that there was no organic problem.

(5) No blame

All activities by family members were seen positively. No person was blamed for what was happening. Each person was seen as trying to sort out a difficult situation. When we stop blaming and accusing we free both ourselves and others to grow. Blame is a hindrance to healing.

(6) Prayer

Throughout this period there were times of protracted and intense prayer. For much of the time, apart from careful listening, the contact had been to pray together. There was nothing that I could offer her other than the support of a listener. She knew her own mind by then, and was gradually learning to trust her own strength and inner voice.

Separation

The immediate result was a separation. With this separation there was also an accompanying reduction in the tension and conflict. Both partners planned for separate homes and began to discuss their futures without mutually attacking each other. There was no attempt on my part to engage them in marital therapy as the invitation and instigation was to come from Harriet. Her husband's depression was reframed as a natural mourning for the loss of a relationship.

Both Harriet and her husband found different homes. Their parenting of the children continued. Harriet discovered many parts of herself which had longed for freedom: the time to be private and the grace of solitude. Her life in the country brought her closer to an understanding of God in all the parts of her life with a changing emphasis from what she 'ought' to be doing to an understanding of what she was being asked to do.

A year later she has been able to meet her husband regularly for a trial period, to talk to him: a period defined by her and acceded to by him. I have found her resolution and persevering faith a remarkable example of healing. She has provided a model for her daughters of how to be resolute without becoming brittle, of courage in her own convictions as a woman, and to be both assertive and compassionate.

Conclusion

I hope that in these brief examples you will have found some glimpse of the healings which have occurred. For each person with whom I have been involved there have been wondrous moments, even in the tears, when we have known the presence of God deeply stirring within us. My life, and that of my family, has been irrevocably touched by the privilege of being involved in the lives of these people. The healing has not been solely theirs. They have taught me about love and perseverance. Beyond that teaching their stories have been used to encourage others. The deaths of George and Sue have not been in vain. They have been a message about hope, about the love of God being manifested in daily life, and the importance of the loving community of the Church coming together to heal.

8 *The Way Forward: A Need for Spiritual Direction*

The main theme of this book has been that, in working together and loving each other, we partake in healing. 'Healing' is used throughout as a verb, rather than as a noun. In this way healing is emphasized as an activity which continues, not something which is static and happens as an isolated event.

This healing activity involves people working together for, and with, each other in the community. The challenge for us as Christians is to widen the boundaries of that community so that we minister not only to ourselves, but to all our neighbours. In the recognition of all people as our neighbours we partake in another realm of healing activity. In some ways each layer of healing is nested one within another. We have our own spiritual journey, yet this journey is often undertaken in the company of others, whether they are our partners, our family or our friends. Similarly, with our friends and families we belong to communities which, like the old tribes, are 'on the move'.

The great challenge we all face now is to combine our own journey with that of those with whom we live. To do so means that we must commune with the Other. When we reach out to the other person we are reaching out to God expressed in that person from the expression of God within ourselves. In this way the body of Christ is coming again. We have the chance now to partake in that body. We become his hands to do his work, his feet to take us to where he is needed, and his voice to bring good news. We are already his heart. When we come together we become of one mind, not losing our individuality, but contributing that individuality to a greater reality. We become more than the sum of our parts: Christ emerges from our merging.

Here again I place the emphasis on the process of coming together. If we can glimpse that reality which involves a simple reaching out towards each other, not a completion which is remote from us, then we can know the 'healing' now.

The wounded healer

An important feature of any healing endeavour is self-awareness. The awareness of 'self' appears to be a difficult concept for Christians as we tend to view self-regard as negative, while focusing on the other person is seen as positive and 'good'. Indeed, throughout this book I have concentrated on service to others. Yet there are dangers involved in such service if we project our own weaknesses on to others without being aware that they arise within us. This reflects the biblical injunction to cast out the mote within our own eye.

Those who care for others often have great difficulty in caring for themselves. Somehow by ministering to the 'weak' using our 'strength', we are actually ministering to our own weaknesses. I know that some people will say that it is not our strength we must work from but the power of the Spirit working within us. I do not believe this helps in any way as it removes us one step further from the area of difficulty, which is that as carers we are relatively incapable of acknowledging the frailties that we seek so assiduously in others. We develop a spiritual or technical armoury to meet the difficulties with which we are faced in our patients or clients, based on a model of being 'gifted' or of having power. The 'power of prayer' doctrine is dangerous if we use it to blind ourselves.

As I have written in an earlier chapter, we can use prayer to keep God out by being too active voicing our own desires. At times we need to be quiet, still, and to listen. The model of powerful healers, of gifted beings, handicaps others if the latter are seen as less powerful, or less gifted. The burden of not being aware of our own weakness is that we cannot express our own needs to our colleagues. Our doubts become submerged and covered up by an aggressive acting out of being 'faithful'. Our sinfulness is hidden beneath a veneer of moral rectitude. Our weakness is disguised by an air of detachment and competency. Eventually this surfaces in our condemnation of the person with whom we are involved. Either we seek them out and 'save them', we blame them for their weakness, or we blame others for not doing enough. They are weak, misguided, helpless and needy. We are strong, filled, powerful and helping, when all the time it is in our own hearts where the problems lie.

Of course caring for the needy, comforting the distressed, and ministering to the sick are central to our healing endeavour. However, what I am advocating is the necessity to be aware of our own needs and our own weaknesses, so that we can truly serve others rather than serving the needs within ourselves through the other person. To do this we must accept our own weaknesses and be willing to admit at times that we are unable to cope, to ask for help and to fail. It is in the seeming weakness and failure that we learn a true compassion.

I believe that it is this unwillingness to acknowledge our own weakness expressed in the desire to be a 'perfect' healer, which lies at the core of our modern concern with 'cure'. Many of the people I see are angry that the counsellors, doctors or helpers they meet only listen to enough of their problem to make a diagnosis of where that problem lies and to come up with a solution. This is the fallacy of being prescriptive. What people ask for is to be listened to first of all, then to be guided to an understanding from which they can act. Prescriptions, medical or spiritual, which are offered prematurely in such situations, are quite inappropriate. Such precocious solutions reflect either the need of the helper to be competent, or a fear which the patient raises within the helper. All too often our very human desire to do something confounds the poverty of our own helplessness.

As counsellors, doctors or healers we have to abdicate this authoritarian position and become partners with those with whom we are involved. This does not mean we abdicate our own authority, rather that we understand that the other person is an authority too. Our task is to bring these two realms of expertise together. But in doing this we cannot expect a 'cure'. God chose what is weak in the world to shame the strong. How many of us faced with a dying patient have searched our textbooks and papers for a better approach, or prayed harder and longer, or looked for friends who have more appropriate gifts, or considered that we are praying for the wrong things, or that perhaps we (or more often the patient) do not have enough faith, when all the time it is our misunderstanding which handicaps us from discovering the truth? And I wonder how many of you already have suggested to yourselves that 'if only I had been a little more spirit-filled, healing would have happened'? How we struggle with our weakness!

What we do by emphasizing cure and perfection is to push the sick, the elderly and the handicapped to the margins of society. We fail to learn from them by being so anxious to change them. Weakness and suffering are important aspects of creative human living which are central to our spiritual teachings. The reification of health, power and strength which negates disability, submission and weakness leads to its own pathology. The poor, weak and ignorant are progressively marginalized. They are treated, patronized, shunned and served but rarely embraced, accepted or acceded to.

Our endeavours must move away from the idea of a 'perfect' health to an understanding of the flawed and wounded healer. Our completion in Christ may only begin to be achieved when we come to understand our own incompleteness.

Spiritual direction

Some of the traps and pitfalls of our own unawareness can be avoided by supervision or spiritual direction. This need not entail the seeking out of some powerful expert who has all the answers. That would be the solution becoming the problem. Rather let us select a colleague with whom we can share our doubts and fears: someone to talk over all the flaws which are raised within us by our work with others. We would also expect of this other person that they would confront us with our own blind spots. The very idea of blind spots is that we cannot see them, not that they exist as dark patches within our field of vision. If we could see the dark patches we would know that we have blind spots. Not only can we 'not see', but most of the time we do not know the extent of our own blindness.

A companion for spiritual direction is also a useful antidote to the notion that we can do it all by ourselves. Occasionally I have tried the route of self-guidance and fallen prey to the trap of self-delusion, and traps of arrogance and spiritual pride which, I might add, I have set and baited myself. When we ask someone else to be involved in our direction we are once more putting into the world the central metaphor that it is in reaching out, in mutuality, that healing and understanding take place.

The recognition and guidance of our failings is not the sole task of the spiritual guide, as this would be an odious task. A far more important task is that of recognizing our gifts. Just as we are blind to our faults we can also be unaware of our gifts. It is our close friends and colleagues who can see the fruits of our work and the evidence of the gifts that we possess.

I am indebted to a seminar led by Clive Calver on the gifts of the Spirit for making this concept explicit. He told the story of his father who had that often overlooked, but supremely important, gift of administration. For years his father had concentrated on developing his gift of evangelism, yet it was his gift for administration which was eventually called from him by colleagues. Through his gift he was able to provide a platform so that others could hear a man who had the gift of evangelism. Surely this is what the gifts of the Spirit are all about, one working with the other to the glory of God. It was through others that the gift was recognized. How often do we ask others what they believe we should be doing in the Church, and if we are using our talents to the full? And how often do we stop to ask them if they have seen evidence of that gift we cherish within ourselves?

The spiritual guide is important. How we choose such a person is partly an artefact of our own spiritual tradition and our own personality. In some traditions the spiritual teacher comes along at precisely the right moment. Others emphasize the need to search for that person, and that the person will have had some training for the task. There is no reason why the spiritual director should be a priest. With the new directions within the Church, and the development of techniques of co-counselling, lay people will have both the experience and the understanding to carry out this task. The mutual aspect of co-counselling has the benefit of a shared journey, yet needs the real vitality of open honesty and trust to avoid a *folie-à-deux*.

Complementary practice and alternative medicine

When the British Medical Association presented a report in 1986 we, as part of the Christian Healing Ministry, were treated as an alternative medical endeavour. By doing so we were placed upon the fringe of healing. Our efforts were seen as peripheral to the scientific healing endeavour within society. While we may be 'comforters', that was to be the extent of our involvement. A staggering feature of that report was the inability of the authors to contemplate any position other than their own, as if healing were the sole prerogative of medicine rather than being a function of many activities within the community. It is to my chagrin that I find Christian groups saying this of other healing endeavours. We treat others in the way we have been treated, rather than doing unto others as we would be done to.

For example, this intolerant attitude is illustrated in the way that acupuncture is treated by some Christian groups. Acupuncture is one of the oldest and most deeply characteristic of the techniques of Chinese medicine. It has been used successfully for over two thousand years to heal a variety of illnesses and malfunctions. Within the past twenty-five years modern western medicine has accommodated some of the techniques and understandings of traditional medicine, and tried to provide a western scientific view of the processes involved. It is important to note that acupuncture is a system of scientific medicine, albeit different from our own, but still scientific. I have heard acupuncture criticized on the grounds that it is founded on an alien spirituality imported from the East. Yet acupuncture makes no such claim for its spiritual antecedents. Similarly modern western medicine, which is so readily embraced by the critics of acupuncture, makes no claim to have a spiritual foundation either.

The Chinese view encapsulated in acupuncture sees the world as a whole in which all the parts are related to each other and also to the whole. There is no creator in this system, no first cause, but a pattern of continually unfolding relationships. The descriptions in this framing of reality do not penetrate to a truth but offer a description of a truth which cannot be grasped. Truth is immanent in everything and is the process itself. Acupuncture refuses to perceive the individual as a microcosm separate from the environment or from the macrocosm.

The criticism of acupuncture is made in ignorance without a real attempt to discover the foundations of the therapy. In the same way we as Christians involved in healing ministries too have been condemned from the basis of ignorance without being truly heard. Listened to, yes; but heard, no. How ironical that we should perpetuate the injustices which we have suffered.

History has a lesson to teach us about the dangers of ignorance and the destruction of knowledge. In the third century BC there was a museum at Alexandria which housed a vast library containing vellums, scrolls and papyri documenting the great works of literature, astronomy, mathematics and medicine. The early works of physicians and physiologists were contained in this library. When Christianity began to take prominence secular knowledge for its own sake was seen as pagan. In AD 390 Bishop

Theophilus destroyed part of the great library. Later, in AD 640 Muslims completed the destruction. Are we to stand in that position today where we destroy rather than understand?

At a recent meeting I was told that it would only be acceptable for Christians to contact alternative practitioners if they asked them about their spiritual beliefs first. I wonder how many of us as Christians do this with our general practitioners? If we did this with our general practitioners, whom we see relatively infrequently, why not extend this questioning to those others who share our daily lives and many of our active health initiatives? Are we really going to quiz our friends and colleagues about the spiritual foundations of their existence, and turn from them if they are not the same as ours? To set ourselves aside from others would be an act which would strike at the heart of our very Christianity. If healing is in acceptance and coming together then we must eschew separation.

The theoretical structure of traditional Chinese medicine has emphasized the balance and harmony between the physical and the psychological aspects of the person. All parts of creation are seen as belonging to an interconnected web of parts. What that system of thought does not acknowledge is the presence of a creator. Yet the understandings of the connectedness of all things are very similar to our Christian understandings of 'though we are many we are one body'. In a similar way Chinese thought stresses the necessity of opposites and the dynamic balance of those opposites. That which is first is seen as being last, and the strong becomes the weak in the constant changing of the world.

The findings of modern physics are beginning to confirm these same understandings. It is these understandings which some Christian writers use to indicate the presence of the Spirit in the world and the way in which everything is connected. The importance of these understandings cannot be ignored. The challenge for us as Christians is how we handle them and apply them in our daily lives and to our theology: a theology which must reflect the present and be applied to the present. This is not to abdicate the Scriptures but to hear them as they speak to us in the light of what we know today.

Acupuncture has nothing to do with parapsychology, occult practice, 'psychic' powers or spiritual forces. It is a system of medical treatment which was present two thousand years before western medicine. There is no need for our present medical or theological chauvinism to dismiss acupuncture. Of course there will be practitioners who make false claims. We cannot eliminate such practitioners from modern medicine, nor can we make claims of such purity within our healing ministries.

Health care

The delivery of primary health care is becoming more ecumenical.

Practitioners are having to face the fact that people are making choices about their own treatment. What they are demanding is time and attention. They need to be heard, to be treated as responsible people, and be given an opportunity to take part in their own health care.

The models of alternative medicine which promote self-care and responsibility, which emphasize wholeness not partiality, are critically important today. Where the problem does lie in alternative or complementary medicine is that in various schools of healing, whether they be alternatively medical or spiritual, there is often no means of establishing accredited practitioners, no supervisory 'college' and no guide to good practice. To establish such supervision would mean a coming together of many practitioners to co-operate in providing such a service. This itself would be healing, but my fear is that the idea is utopian.

Modern western medicine has the benefit of humility in its own tradition, in that at the heart of science there is always the readiness to doubt and to accept that current knowledge will be overturned. Perhaps many of its practitioners or proponents forget that. Furthermore, there are standards of scrutiny and practice embedded in the medical system. When we come to scrutinize alternative practice that structure cannot always be discerned. Christian healing may also be part of that realm of complementary practice where a structure cannot be as readily discerned. We cannot offer that structure other than within the body of a Church.

Conclusion

Healing raises many of the issues confronting Christianity today. First, it challenges us all to go out into the world and act as Christians. Second, it demands a co-operation between laity and clergy in the promotion and maintenance of our corporate health. We belong to a royal priesthood of all believers and to this we are all called. The injunction of Christ is to go out, teach and heal. Third, we are all encouraged to use our talents without personal exception in reaching out to others. Expertise is valued, but in a role of facilitation. The expertise of all persons is promoted. Christian healing has no academy or college with lauded graduates. Fourth, there are no barriers to healing: we must reach out to all our neighbours. In recognizing all people as our neighbours then we further promote healing in the world.

If we take up healing then we must accept that our theology will be challenged. The administration of the sacraments of healing will raise implications for the administration of the sacrament of the Eucharist. The involvement of laity will raise the issue of roles within the Church. The growing involvement of women in the healing ministry will also continue the move towards the ordination of women. It will be a mark of our faith and love that we do not, in the pursuit of healing, promote division. The world is hungry, and we are part of that hunger. The world is in need and we are that need. In our hands we have the capacity to clench our fists or to hold out our palms. The choice is with us in every moment of human life. The time to begin is now. Look to the person on your right and reach out to them. Look to the person on your left and reach out to them. It is as simple as that!

Bibliography

Healing

There are many books on healing. The following titles are a useful introduction to practice.

Cosslett, N., *His Healing Hands*. Hodder and Stoughton, London 1985.

England, A., *We Believe in Healing*. Marshalls, London 1982.

Foster, R., *Celebration of Discipline*. Hodder and Stoughton, London 1980.

Lawrence, R., *Invitation to Healing*. Kingsway, Eastbourne 1979.

Linn, M., Linn, D., and Fabricant, S., *Prayer Course for Healing Life's Hurts*. Paulist Press, New York 1983.

McNutt, F., *Healing*. Bantam 1974.

Maddocks, M., *The Christian Healing Ministry*. SPCK, London 1981.

Maddocks, M., *Journey to Wholeness*. Triangle, London 1986.

Complementary medicine

Fulder, S., *The Handbook of Complementary Medicine*. Coronet, London 1984.

Inglis, B., *Natural Medicine*. Fontana, Glasgow 1979.

Inglis, B., and West, R., *The Alternative Health Guide*. Michael Joseph, London 1983.

Kaptchuk, T., *Chinese Medicine*. Rider, London 1983.

King, F., *Rudolf Steiner and Holistic Medicine*. Rider, London 1986.

Pietroni, P., *Holistic Living*. Dent, London 1986.

Salmon, J., *Alternative Medicines*. Tavistock, London 1984.

Background material

Bateson, G., *Mind and Nature*. Fontana, Glasgow 1979.

Bateson, G., *Steps to an Ecology of Mind*. Paladin, London 1973.

Capra, F., *The Tao of Physics*. Fontana, Glasgow 1975.

Cupitt, D., *The Sea of Faith*. BBC, London 1985.

Dossey, L., *Space, Time and Medicine*. RKP, London 1982.

Koestler, A., *Janus: A Summing Up*. Picador, London 1979.

Papers by the author

Aldridge, D. (1987), 'Families, cancer and dying', *Family Practice* (in press).

Aldridge, D., and Pietroni, P. C. P. (1987), 'The clinical assessment of acupuncture for asthma therapy' *Journal of the Royal Society of Medicine*, 80(4); 222–4.

Aldridge, D. (1986), 'Methods of assessment: The measurement of effects and their differences'. In Pietroni *et al.* (eds), *Report on the B.M.A. Board of Science Working Party on Alternative Therapy*, London, British Holistic Medical Association, pp. 50–57.

Aldridge, D. (1986), 'The delivery of primary health care; general practice and complementary approaches to health care', *Holistic Health*, 12: 32–5.

Aldridge, D. (1986), 'Licence to heal', *Crucible*, April/June: 58–66.

Aldridge, D. (1985), 'Stress; the questionnaire results', *Holistic Health*, 7: 12–15.

Aldridge, D. (1985), 'Children in distress', *Crucible*, April/June: 67–76.

Aldridge, D. (1984), 'Suicidal behaviour and family interaction; a brief review', *Journal of Family Therapy*, 6: 309–22.

Aldridge, D., and Dallos, R. (1986), 'Distinguishing families where suicidal behaviour is present from families where suicidal behaviour is absent', *Journal of Family Therapy*, 8: 243–52.

Aldridge, D., and Rossiter, J. (1985), 'Difficult patients, intractable symptoms and spontaneous recovery in suicidal behaviour', *Journal of Systemic and Strategic Therapies*, 4.3: 66–76.

Aldridge, D., and Rossiter, J. (1984), 'A strategic assessment of deliberate self-harm', *Journal of Family Therapy*, 6: 119–32.

Aldridge, D., and Rossiter, J. (1983), 'A strategic approach to suicidal behaviour', *Journal of Systemic and Strategic Therapies*, 2(4): 49–62.

Dallos, R., and Aldridge, D. (1987), 'Handing it on: family constructs, symptoms and choice', *Journal of Family Therapy* (in press).

Dallos, R., and Aldridge, D. (1986), 'Change: How do we recognise it?' *Journal of Family Therapy*, 8: 45–59.

Pietroni, P. C., and Aldridge, D. (1986), Summary of Discussion on BMA Report, *Holistic Medicine*, 1.

Useful Addresses

Organizations

The following organizations will direct you to people in your local area and also supply further resources.

The ACORN TRUST, Whitehill Chase, High Street, Bordon, Hampshire. This trust has a house which is used as an administrative headquarters, a training resource, and a healing centre. The organization promotes the co-operation of medicine and the Church. There is a list of local advice centres and an introductory training course for counsellors called Christian Listeners.

The CHURCHES COUNCIL FOR HEALTH AND HEALING, 17 Marylebone Road, London NW1 5LT. The council has been established for a long time. It is very broadly based and ecumenical. There are training courses and a vast amount of co-ordinated information about other organizations.

The BRITISH HOLISTIC MEDICAL ASSOCIATION, 79 Gloucester Place, London NW1 6DX. This organization has comprehensive information on holistic and complementary medicine; educational activities; reading lists, a newsletter and a journal; and a list of local practitioners.

Further help

The BRITISH ASSOCIATION FOR COUNSELLING, 37a Sheep Street, Rugby, Warwickshire, publish a directory of counselling agencies and organizations edited by Antony Clayton.

Index